D1546246

Mind & Mend Your Hips

Better Hip Health

Learn how to improve your hip health, prepare for and recover from hip surgery, and improve your overall movement through the Alexander Technique.

Ann Rodiger,
M.AmSAT, RSME

Ann Rodiger

Founder and Director

Balance Arts Center

151 W. 30th St. Floor 3

New York City, New York, 10001

USA

www.balanceartscenter.com

Print ISBN: 978-1-66784-331-5

eBook ISBN: 978-1-66784-332-2

This book is printed on acid-free paper.

This book is not intended to substitute for medical consultation, advice or treatment. The author and publisher disclaim any and all liability arising directly or indirectly from the use of any information contained in this book.

Edited by Liz Gessner, Cover design, graphics, and layout by Morgan Van Gele.

Acknowledgements

As the founder and director of the Balance Arts Center (BAC) in New York City, which I founded in 2008, I teach the Alexander Technique (AT) and diverse programs, including an AT Teacher Training course.[1] My work has evolved from the analytic, movement, and pedagogical systems of Frederick Matthias Alexander and Rudolf Laban. I am grateful to Alexander and Laban for their contributions which have guided me and become the central focus of my life and work.

Alexander's method teaches fundamental movement theory and a process for change that can be applied to our movement in all situations. Laban created a structure for movement observation, exploration, analysis, and description. Together, both these frameworks foster a profound understanding of how we think about and experience ourselves in environments with which we interact.

The work of Raymond Dart and Irmgard Bartenieff inform the movement laboratory work we do at the Balance Arts Center.

---

1   The Alexander Technique Teacher Training is a 1,600-hour course completed during a period of 3-5 years.

Both modalities address fundamental and developmental aspects of movement.

I would like to acknowledge the training I received in the Alexander Technique from Joan and Alex Murray while they were in Urbana, Illinois. I was fortunate to be a student in their very first AT teacher training program.[2]

I am also grateful to Dr. Steven Stuchin, an orthopedic surgeon for hips and hands, for his expert knowledge and talent as a surgeon. His surgical gifts and wonderful bedside manner made both of my hip surgeries a positive experience.

Thank you to the friends and family who helped me through my time in the hospital and who have continued to support me throughout my full recovery.

Lastly, I want to thank Liz Gessner, Morgan Van Gele, Jessica Goldring, Thomas Baird, Carol Boggs, Cate Deicher, N. Alana Risser, and the staff and students at the Balance Arts Center, including Alice MacDonald, Lindy Rogers, Nathan Are, Kari Ostensen, Allie Kronick, and Surabhee Arjunwadkar, for their contributions, support, and encouragement in the writing of this book.

---

2   I trained with Joan and Alex Murray in Urbana, Illinois. Joan Murray was a
     dancer and understood the demands the profession puts on one's body. Through
     the sustained study of their training course, I found improved coordination,
     connection, and awareness.

Contents

Videos

https://www.balanceartscenter.com/

mind-and-mend-your-hips-videos

A journey of 1,000 miles begins with a single step.

Tao Te Ching by Laozi

Notes to the Reader

As of the writing of this book, I have had both hips replaced. The Alexander Technique has given me the tools and awareness with which to prepare for and support my surgeries and make a full recovery. As a teacher of the Alexander Technique, I have also worked with many students with hip issues. Some have needed surgery while others have been able to resolve their issues through better use. I present concepts through the lens of a patient, student and teacher in the hope that you, too, may benefit from the Alexander Technique in your journey to optimal hip health.[3]

This book begins by exploring the fundamental concepts of the Alexander Technique. We will look at the elements of movement, posture, and habit, and examine how integrating an awareness of these elements can change our lives. From there, you can begin to perceive the choices available to you and how

---

3   For more on those who have influenced my understanding of the AT, see
     Appendix V.

you might choose differently in order to develop better balance and coordination.

These fundamental Alexander Technique concepts are applicable to your whole body and all of your movement at any time. Working with these concepts can become a gateway to connection with a greater sense of self, continually deepening and even becoming a lifelong pursuit.

If you have picked up this book because you are experiencing hip pain but have no need at this point for surgery, it can serve as a guide for how to minimize pain and develop better hip health habits. If you are post hip surgery, the information here can support and even improve your recovery. For those readers who are headed for hip surgery, this book walks you through every step of the process, from finding the right doctor to rediscovering a life of freedom in movement.

How to Use This Book

This book functions as both a reference book and a step-by-step guide. Take a moment at the start to browse through and see what information or sections catch your attention. This may be where you want to begin. For instance, if you are using a cane or a walker, you might want to read ahead to instructions on how to do this properly, before you tackle the more fundamental principles introduced at the beginning of the book.

Ultimately, start at the beginning and build from there. The first eight chapters present information incrementally so that you can learn to connect your thinking with your movement in an increasingly clear way. If at any point, you feel you are losing that sense of connection, you can return to the earlier exercises and reset.

One way to get the most out of this book is to assume an attitude of possibility and self-discovery. We learn best when we get curious and are willing to explore, when we allow ourselves to have fun. When we can *just play* without any pressure to achieve a goal and let go of any judgment, we free ourselves to discover things we would otherwise never find. As you move through this book, you will be invited—through a series of Awareness Building and Movement Activities—to notice what you notice and direct yourself. Remember, awareness of any sensory mode is useful. You are practicing the act of paying attention and becoming aware of how your mind and movement influence each other. I suggest you see *what happens* and *have a go* at the ideas and activities. Any response is welcome and you might find yourself completely surprised.

Lasting change comes from an accumulation of small, incremental, and sustained shifts in attention. It is important to honor each step of this process and know that you are moving toward your potential, even if at times you may feel like you are going backwards. This work is delicate, nuanced, and often more about having a new thought than it is about taking any remedial action. Staying with the investigation through consistent practice will bring you to a new level of awareness from which balance and flow will unfold.

My favorite teaching experiences are the "ah-ha" moments when students discover and embody new ideas and experiences. It is my hope that this book will bring you many "ah-ha" moments!

CHAPTER 1

Discovering the Whole – Unified Field of Awareness

We will start by exploring the fundamental concepts of the Alexander Technique, looking at the elements of movement, posture and habit, and examining how integrating a sense of awareness into everything we do can change our lives.

First, we will look at how your mind and body function together when you are in motion. Developing an understanding of how they interact develops self-agency and will provide a baseline from which you can start shifting habits of thought and movement in order to improve your hip health.

If you are experiencing hip pain, something has gone awry. Learning how to self-reflect in order to direct yourself into better balance is the first step. Refining our movements requires that we first become aware of our thoughts and identify the elements of the whole. From there, we can begin to explore how to integrate them into our *Unified Field of Awareness.*

As we explore these ideas, we will apply them to activities related to the hips and walking. The goal is to embody the process of attending to and directing yourself so that paying attention to the whole becomes habitual.

Unified Field of Awareness[4]

Unified Field of Awareness includes our thoughts, emotions, and senses as well as our perception of space and time. We each develop our own unique patterns of awareness as we move through our daily lives, frequently favoring one sense over others. You may be someone who prefers to *see,* while someone else may rely on their keen sense of smell. Some people are very tuned into how their body moves in space while others have little awareness of these kinesthetic and proprioceptive sensibilities. One is not better than another; these are all important and valuable ways of experiencing the world. What is important is

---

4   The term *Unified Field of* Awareness is generally attributed to Frank Pierce Jones (1905-1975), although he may not have put the phrase together per se. It is a term widely adopted in Alexander Technique teaching and discussions. Jones, a Classics professor at Brown University, studied the AT with Alexander and his brother A.R., taught the AT himself, and researched and wrote extensively about the Technique. His main writing is entitled *Freedom to Change, The Development and Science of the Alexander Technique* first published in 1976 under the title *Body Awareness in Action.* The book is now available from Mouritz.

identifying your preference and understanding how they relate to what is going on in your body.

Familiarizing ourselves with the multiple elements of our awareness allows us to access all of them as needed. In the Awareness Building exercise that follows, work with the sequences, paying attention to where your mind goes. See if you begin to notice your individual preferences.

Awareness Building
Field of Awareness Exploration

Start by noticing which of the following you are most aware of:

- Sound

- Light

- Color

- Smell

- Temperature

- Air flow

- Space around you

- Vibrations in the space, vocal or otherwise

- Tactile stimulus

- Emotion

- Taste

- Bodily sensation

- Your weight on the ground

- Your response to gravity

- Amount of force you are using to do an activity

- Your own internal space

With this sense of where your awareness goes, explore the following sequences while either standing or sitting. Take your time. Be sure to notice each sensory perception before moving on to the next.

Sequence 1:

- Focus on the sounds around you.

- Now, add sight to that awareness.

- Add the air temperature to your awareness.

- Add the smells in the room to your awareness.

- Add a sense of your weight on the ground.

Reset and start again.

Sequence 2:

- Sense your body weight as it contacts the ground or the chair.

- Take in the space of the room.

- Add your sense of smell to your sense of space.

- Add your sense of sight to this awareness.

- Now, add hearing.

- Feel the texture of your clothes against your skin. Add this to your awareness.

Take these explorations of your awareness with you as you go about your day. Notice how and where your attention moves. Which forms of perception do you access more readily? Practice adding other senses to your field of awareness until you can attend to multiple sources of input, simultaneously.

Your Attention Within the *Unified Field of Awareness*

Your attention is how, when, and where you interface with your *Unified Field of Awareness*. One of the main tenets of AT is self-agency, how we are able to direct our thinking and in so doing, direct the way we move and where our attention goes. This occurs in two parts. The first step is becoming aware of our thoughts. This is called attending to our thoughts. Once we are aware of what we are thinking, the second step is to choose to continue with useful thoughts and let the rest go. This process is fundamental to improving your body in motion. It means taking yourself off "automatic pilot" and from there, slowing down and giving yourself more time between thoughts and action.

Doing this can be very revealing. We often think the way things are is the only way they can be, that the way our body works and moves is fixed and there are no other options. As we slow down, we create the space to become aware of these underlying assumptions. Recognizing our thoughts, we can evaluate them and choose to focus on the ones that are accurate and most beneficial. This self-agency enables us to change a situation.

If you are having hip issues, this slowing down in order to cultivate awareness may initially heighten your discomfort. Your instinct might be to adjust yourself to lessen the pain. That might mean hiking up one hip, leaning to one side, or stiffening your leg. This is an opportunity to take note of how you are compensating.

The Movement Activity below allows you to explore how your thinking affects your movement. While applicable to the body-mind interface in general, it is a particularly useful place to start if you are dealing with hip issues.

Movement Activity
Thinking Affects Your Movement

Start sitting.

Think of your body as being heavy and stiff, as if it is made of concrete or filled with rocks.

- Maintaining this sense of heaviness, come to standing.

- What do you notice?

- Sit down.

- Now, think of your body as light, buoyant, and airy.

- Sustaining this sense of lightness, come to standing.

- What do you notice?

- How was your experience of standing when you felt light different from your experience of standing when you felt heavy?

- Remember there is no right or wrong. Every observation is important and valuable.

This is another exercise that can help you see how your thinking affects your sensory experience. Notice what emerges in your awareness as you play with this spatial experiment.

Awareness Building
Spatial Thinking

As you move around your space, notice what you sense as you allow your whole body to take on the property of:

- A paper doll

- A cube

- A sphere

- A sphere collapsing in on itself

- A sphere exploding outward

- A sphere made of wood

- A sphere made of water

- A sphere suspended in the space

Your Whole Body

One of the most fundamental concepts in AT is that your whole body is participating in everything you do. Although some parts may be moving through space more actively than others, your body serves you best when your entire structure is able to move in response to an activity. For example, if you move your arm forward and allow the rest of the body to respond as counterbalance, you discover a flow of energy. Instead, if you stiffen, keeping the rest of your body still, you are resisting the body's natural response to provide counterbalance. In doing so, you cause a restriction which blocks the vital flow of your energy.

It is also important to know that even when you are not in motion, your body has a constant vitality created by muscular tone and energy moving through you. This continuous support system provides a constant baseline from which you are always functioning. What is often misunderstood is that with conscious awareness, we can shift that baseline to a level that allows for greater balance and ease.

Finding and cultivating optimal tone and flow is essential even when your attention is being pulled to your hip's impingement on your structure. Becoming aware of and beginning to allow for this ultimate balancing will not only help to alleviate current discomfort, but it will also begin your process of healing.

Dimensionality – Volume

Your body is an omnidimensional structure that contains multidimensional pulls moving simultaneously in oppositional directions. When it comes to spatial awareness, we all know up-down, down-up, left-right, right-left, and side-side. These fundamental dimensions of *length*, *width*, and *depth* are just a starting point. There are countless other oppositions at play (for example, running on the diagonal), constantly moving towards, through, and beyond our physical structure.

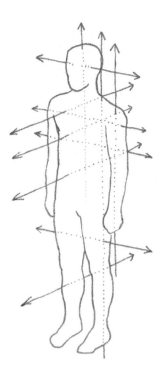

Fig. 1
The Three Fundamental Dimensions: Length, Width, and Depth

These pulls are forces of nature that support you as they move through you. They have an inherent balance that creates your body's own unique arrangement and volume. When there is an interference, and one dimension becomes overemphasized at the expense of the others, the overall balance is disturbed. We often over-lengthen our body in an effort to appear taller, and end up compromising our width and depth which narrows our structure and diminishes the amount of support we have available. For those with hip issues, the interference occurs at the hip joint impeding the energetic flow of these directions.

Awareness Building
Dimensionality

Here are some activities to help you explore your dimensionality. They can be done sitting, standing, or lying down.

Length—your distance up to down—is your dominant dimension. Here are ways to sense your length:

- Sense the distance from the top of your head to the soles of your feet. Then sense the distance from the soles of your feet to the top of your head.

- Bring your attention to your breath, allowing the sensation of your airflow to move along your length.

- Keep track of this length now as you both inhale and exhale.

- Now, extend this sense of length beyond your body's boundary in both directions, past the top of your head and down into the ground.

Width—your breadth from side to side—is your secondary dimension. Here are ways to sense your width:

- Place your arms at your sides. Sense the distance from the outside of your left arm through your torso to outside of your right arm.

- Move your awareness down and notice the continuation of this expanse as it extends from one hand to the other.

- Inhale and notice how the breadth of your ribcage increases. Maintain that width as you exhale.

- Allow this sense of width to extend beyond your body's boundary.

Depth—your distance from front to back—is the third dimension, filling out your dimensionality. Here are ways to sense your depth:

- Notice the distance between your nose and the back of your head.

- Notice the distance between your sternum and your spine.

- Notice the distance between your pubic bone and tailbone.

- Allow this sense of depth in these areas to extend beyond your body's boundary.

Biotensegrity and *Suspension*

Let's take this concept of dimensionality and volume a step further. What happens when you consider your whole body not as a static container but as a suspension system with its own dynamic volume? How does it feel to trust that the inherent dynamics of your structure will support you?

You have just started to explore the concepts of *biotensegrity* and suspension. Developing an awareness of these forces will allow you to change how you use your body.

It is worth taking a minute to correct a common misconception. Our skeletal system is not an arrangement of bone-on-bone. In fact, our bones exist in a suspension with various viscous fluids acting as padding between them. Rather than thinking of the traditional skeleton, think of an X-ray in which the bones appear to be floating.

Once you have factored in this sense of cushioning, you can see your structure as a gentle push and pull of forces in which the bones and organs are suspended in a delicate balance. You can then think of the support coming from the muscles, tendons, and ligaments: "guy wires" toned to provide stability to an otherwise free-form structure.

Entertaining this concept of *biotensegrity* in which the struts do not touch each other is a paradigm shift for many of us. We no longer think of our bodies as bones piled on top of each other (the post-and-beam or stack-of-bricks system) but as a form that is fluid and mobile. Play with the figures below to begin revising how you experience your body. Start by allowing yourself, for just a moment, to experience a state of collapse.

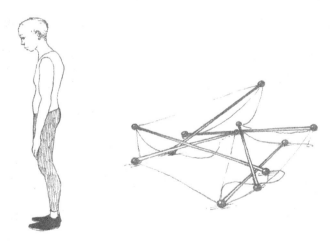

Fig. 2
Compromised Biotensegrity Model

The loss of suspension shown in the toy model in Fig. 2 results in a compromised form which then compresses and obstructs the volume. The struts are still there but the connecting links have lost their tone and gone relatively lax. Similarly, a collapsed posture occurs when the body's musculature lacks appropriate tone and/or the ligaments are overstretched. Both structures in Fig. 2 have lost their spring and resilience.

Next, let's play with shifting into a state of appropriate tone. Notice in Fig. 3 how the toy model is in its full form, upright and dimensional. The human model is upright and balanced, as well. Move yourself now into this more suspended posture. Rather than just pulling yourself upright, think of finding suspension by reinitiating your volume and dimensionality. Do you notice a change in your breathing? What else emerges?

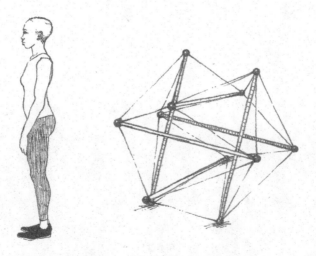

Fig. 3
Optimal Biotensegrity Model

Let's stay with this concept a little longer. If you happen to have your own tensegrity model, pinch it on one side. Notice how even though some of it still appears buoyant, the stress throughout the structure is now uneven. This loss of equipoise compromises the structure's stability. This same principle applies to the body. When our *biotensegrity* system is compromised—for example, by a bone-on-bone hip condition—we become physically restricted and less able to find our dynamic balance.[5]

One of the ways to meet the restrictions of your current condition (and prepare yourself for post-surgery, if that is your way forward) is to see yourself as a pinched version of the *biotensegrity* model. From there, you can direct your awareness to reinitiate as much dimensionality and suspension as is available to you. Consciously cultivating this spatial way of thinking allows you to find the easiest and most dynamically responsive organization of your structure.

Exploring Gravity and Ground Reaction Force (GRF)

Our bodies in space are at any moment responding to a layering of forces. Adding on to the concepts of *biotensegrity* and suspension, we must next explore the role of gravity as it interacts with the body.

---

5   If you would like to build your own tensegrity toy there are instructions at carolboggs.com. It is a fun project to do and I have seen students have big "ah-ha" moments at the end of the project.

Newton states in his third law of motion that when force is exerted on an object, the object exerts an equal force in the opposite direction. Think of a baseball: a 95 m/ph pitch once hit travels at a rate of speed and in a direction opposite and proportional to the force and direction it meets in the bat. Think, too, of a swimmer pushing off a pool wall. It is the push into the wall that allows the swimmer to accelerate back through the water in the opposite direction.

In the case of the body, Newton's law of motion applies all the time, whether we are horizontal or vertical. When we are vertical, the oppositional force is a rebounding motion that travels up through us. We contact the ground not only while standing or walking, but also when sitting on a chair or on a bicycle. In any of these circumstances, if we allow for that oppositional push to move through us, we can experience an upward direction which will allow for our body to have its optimal tensegrity. Basically, we need to get out of the way so that the natural forces may be distributed evenly throughout our structure.

We all are aware of gravity as the constant pulling of our bodies toward the center of the earth. What may not be so obvious is the equal and opposite force moving away from the earth's center. This oppositional response to gravity is known as the Ground Reaction Force (GRF). It is the energy of the *rebound* and can be felt as a flow moving up through our bodies. The work we are here to do is to learn how we can better allow this force to flow through our own bodies.

Our job is to use our thinking and awareness to optimize the GRF. The more we eliminate interference, the more we can recruit the GRF's dynamic energy to more fully support our system.

In the Alexander Technique, some teachers when referring to the GRF will direct a student to "go up". This can be effective as long as the student does not pull on themselves or actually try *to do* anything. It is about releasing and allowing. Even the subtlest upward pulling can cause stiffness and reduced movement options. The GRF is strong and when allowed, provides a sense of lightness, fuller breathing, and ease of movement.

First, we will explore the GRF in a general way. This is the first of the Movement Activities that is accompanied by a video. You are strongly encouraged to watch the accompanying videos as they bring the words on these pages to life.

Movement Activity
Gravity and Ground Reaction Force

(Video #1: Hi-Bounce Ball and Bean Bag)

This activity explores gravity and the GRF. It is meant to let you experience the rebound of the GRF that you may already sense in your body. You will need a hi-bouncing ball and a bean bag (or a book).

Activity:

- Drop the bean bag or book on the floor and notice if it bounces.

- Now, bounce the ball and notice the difference.

- Next, bounce the ball and follow the ball's bounce with your hand. You can keep the bounce going by adding a little pressure to the ball as it goes back down towards the ground.

- Keep the ball bouncing continuously and with the palm of your hand, start to follow the ball on its upward trajectory. Allow your palm to sense the ball's moment of suspension just before it reverses direction and heads back to the floor.

- Play with this and see how it feels in your body when you ride the ball's movement with your hand.

Now, tune into this sense of flow and buoyancy in your whole body by feeling gravity and the GRF moving in tandem throughout your whole structure:

- Start by noticing where your body is contacting the ground. If you are sitting, notice where you are contacting your chair.

- Sense gravity pulling you toward the earth's center.

- Add to this sensation an awareness of an opposite force: the push of the GRF coming up through the body.

- Have the thought that you can experience both directions simultaneously.

- Give yourself time to feel this subtle exchange and know you can come back to this activity as often as necessary.

This practice of tuning into your flow and buoyancy is something you can do anytime, anywhere, as often as you like. Fully experiencing this concept means allowing yourself to notice that you are constantly coming in and out of a delicate equilibrium.

The more sensitive you become to this subtle ongoing motion, the more you can tap into your own flow.

Dynamic Balance

Dynamic balance is maintained by the body's musculature continuously adapting to and recalibrating its tone. When your whole body is allowed to respond to each moving part at every moment, you are in a state of optimal balance where your body is able to be fully responsive to the actions you are asking it to do.

Think of the toy tensegrity model in its full suspension. Our body in dynamic balance is this tensegrity structure in action, its entirety responding to every small movement it encounters. The following exercise allows you to embody this concept and play with further refining your sense of dynamic balance.

Movement Activity
Dynamic Balance

(Video #2: Dynamic Balance)

This activity allows you to experience how subtle movements of your eyes and head can affect the balance of your whole body.

- Sit on your sit bones with your easiest balance and best alignment.

- Let your feet be flat on the floor, hip-width apart, at a comfortable distance in front of you.

- Allow your head to balance on your spine so that you are looking straight ahead.

- Now from this position of equilibrium, allow your eyes to make the small movements necessary for you to look toward your knees.

- Notice how your head follows your eye movement. Refine this movement so that you are moving from the very top of your spine.

- Breathe.

- Notice that when you allow your body to dynamically respond to this eye movement, your pelvis responds by rocking slightly back on your sit bones.

- Raise your eyes back up to look forward again. Allow your body, including your pelvis, to respond, readjusting back to the vertical.

- Next, look to your left. Allow your whole head, neck, and back to respond to this eye movement.

- Come back to center. Now, look to your right.

- Play with this activity, looking in different directions and noticing what effect moving one body part has on the whole.

Becoming aware of how your whole body is involved in every movement may at first seem tiring and unnecessary. By working with this activity, you can begin to see that holding or bracing one part of your body causes you to potentially lose your sense of flow. Allowing your whole structure to be involved in this tensegrous way (regardless of the size, speed or type of movement in which you engage), sustains your connection to the ground and the GRF, allowing the dynamic balance to occur throughout your body.

Compensations

When there is interference of any kind with the flow—for example, an overly tight muscle resulting from a tension habit or a structural issue such as a bone-on-bone hip joint, we develop ways of working around the limitation. These work-arounds happen when one part (or parts) takes on the function of another part (or parts). These "compensations" are useful as they keep us functioning and in motion.

Think about what happens in your body when you stub your toe or twist your ankle. You don't want to put weight on that foot. Quickly, your entire body becomes affected. You might sense fatigue in your back, your other leg may feel strained. You may stiffen your jaw in reaction to the pain, even though that part of you is quite far away from the site of your injury.

If the hip joint has become painful and your movement feels at all restricted, you are likely compensating in some way. You may be lifting the side of your pelvis up to bring your leg through. Or swiveling the pelvis forward on the restricted side. You may be limping or listing (tilting) to one side with the whole torso. Whatever your form of compensation, you are responding to the loss of fluid movement of your hip socket.

Work-arounds put stress and strain on the opposite hip, sacroiliac joints, knees, and ankles as well as the head, neck, and back. They can sneak up on us, appearing gradually, and even going unnoticed at first. They usually start with us telling ourselves things like, "I know I'm leaning over but it is just a little bit. It will only happen this time."

It is important to recognize compensations as they emerge and monitor their progression. Failing to do so risks them becoming habitual. Over time as an obstruction increases in intensity, compensations tend to both accumulate and become normalized. When this happens, we may begin to see our work-arounds as our only option for movement.

Thinking about the relationship of one part of your body to another will help you understand how compensations affect your whole structure. In the activity below, you are asked to deliberately create an interference in your body structure. The interference and resulting compensation can be obvious or subtle. As you play with this concept of interference and compensation, notice what comes into your awareness.

Movement Activity
Compensations

(Video #3: Compensations)

This activity is an opportunity to see how your whole body responds when one part is restricted.

- Move your left shoulder and notice what you sense in your right hip.

- Move your right hip and notice what you sense in your left shoulder.

- Keep your left shoulder still while you move the rest of your body. What do you notice?

- Now stand up and begin to walk. Lead your movement with your pelvis and notice what happens in your chest.

- Continue walking, now turning one leg and foot outward. How does your body respond?

- Take a shorter stride with your right leg. What do you notice?

- Walk forward leading with one hip. Notice how the rest of your body responds.

- Now, exaggerate the movement of your right shoulder. Notice what happens with your left hip.

- Next, keep your right hip from bending as you walk. What do you experience?

Throughout this activity, you were experimenting with the effect interference has on your *biotensegral* system. As you can see, if something is dominating your attention, you may be pulled to focus mainly on that body part. The temptation may be to set about "fixing" or "controlling" that part. It is, however, essential to keep track of the bigger picture—your thinking as well as your whole body in motion and the space around you. For those with hip concerns, this practice will enable you to better support your hip joint. Rather than trying to fix the impingement, focus instead on the movement as it is occurring in your full body.

CHAPTER 2

Developing an Accurate
Body Image

The next step in the awareness building process is creating an accurate mental map of the body's structure, how the parts of the body exist in relationship to each other. We touched on this in Chapter 1 in the discussion of how bones do not rest on other bones but exist in a vital suspension system. This chapter will focus on how developing a more accurate mental image of your internal structure can more fully inform how you experience your body in motion. Appreciating how each part fits into the whole *biotensegral* structure will allow you a new understanding and greater awareness from which to initiate all your movements.

We all have a sense of our body-part locations and where movement occurs whether we are conscious of it or not. When these images and sensory experiences are accurate and clear, we direct ourselves in a useful manner. When our images are inaccurate or unclear, we send faulty messages to the wrong locations.

To use an increasingly outdated analogy, if a phone wire is not going to the right location or you have dialed the wrong number, your message won't reach the intended recipient. Similarly, an inaccurate map of your body parts, how they fit and move together, causes you to send signals to wrong locations. You don't have to be an expert anatomist to appreciate this concept. Developing a proper awareness of your anatomical structure and a refined attunement to your sensory experience are essential tools in your search for greater ease of movement.

Head and Neck

The head and neck are a great place to start when trying to understand how an accurate body image impacts your functioning. Where you think your head balances on your spine affects how you manage the weight of your head in relation to your entire body. It also affects the blood flow and nervous impulses from your body through your neck to your brain.

For example, if you think your head attaches to your spine at the vertebrae at the level of the bottom of your jaw, you will be sending the message to move your head at a location that is too low. Moving from that lower vertebra puts extra stress and pressure on a joint that is not intended to perform that function. That vertebra is one in a series of joints intended to form the natural curve in your neck meant to connect to your skull.

Movement of the head and neck is meant to mainly occur higher up, at the very top of your spine. Close your eyes imagining the space that is between and slightly below your ears. You can also touch this space with your fingers. Open your eyes, look down toward your knees, and move your head from this space. This is moving from the top of your spine. Moving your head from here allows you to more easily release the downward pressure your 10-12 pound head puts on your body. It also frees up your entire body to respond to the natural bounce of the GRF.

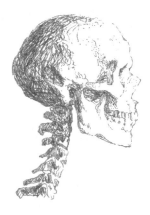

Fig. 4
Head on Spine

This next activity encourages you to explore the dimensions of your head beyond the two-dimensional flat surface you see when looking at yourself in the mirror. As you play with the ideas below, and watch the accompanying video, you may discover that your head has a volume and depth you had not tuned into before, and that you also have a longer neck than you ever imagined.

Awareness Building
Head and Neck

(Video #4: Head and Neck)

Below is a list of aspects of the dimensionality of your head and neck. Notice these, first, in Fig. 4 above. Then sense them in your own body. Take your time with each aspect. Feel free to use your hands to more clearly perceive each point on this map of your head and neck.

- Your neck has a subtle natural forward curve.

- Your neck comes all the way up behind your jaw and nose.

- A significant portion of your head is above your eyes.

- Your jaw is only attached to your skull, not to your spine.

- There is space between your jaw and spine.

- Your head is both in front of and behind the balance point on your spine.

- The back of your skull acts as a counterbalance to your face.

Head, Neck, and Back (HNB)

Let's add your back to the map. The HNB relationship is the primary structure of your body. It houses your brain, spinal cord, and vital organs and is the central location to which your appendages connect and move through. In short, it forms the foundation for all the movements you do.

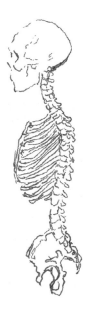

Fig. 5
Head, Neck, and Back

This next activity expands your awareness of your body's dimensionality to include the back as well as the head and neck. As you play with the ideas below, and watch the accompanying video, you may begin to discover the potential you possess for movement between the head and the pelvis—the two ends of your spine.

Awareness Building
Head, Neck, and Back

(Video #5: Head, Neck, and Back)

Below is a list of aspects of your dimensionality from head to tail. Again, notice these, first, in the image above. As you begin to sense them in your body, take your time and use your hands to help you expand your perception.

- Like your skull on your spine, your HNB has length, width, and depth.

- There is distance connecting the top of your head to the bottom of your spine.

- The subtle forward curve of your neck is complemented by two more curves, one in the chest and one in the lower back.

- Your torso has depth.

- The spine is housed in the back half of your torso.

- The bottom of the sternum slants up toward the back of your head.

- The ribs are not horizontal but slant down from the spine and then wrap upwards in front towards the sternum.
- There is space between your ribs and pelvis.
- The pelvis also has length, width, and depth.
- The spine is included in the back of the pelvis.

Arms

Before we address the hip-pelvis-leg connection, we need to take a moment to look at the arms. What do my arms have to do with my hips, you might ask. Everything! As an extension of the HNB system, the arms, while used for more refined movements than the legs, are part of the *biotensegrity* structure. Because of this, how we use our arms directly affects our hips.

When we allow the joints of our arms to move and participate appropriately in our activities, they are able to support our overall balance and flow. What we will look at now is how to monitor the ease and fluidity with which you use your arms. In so doing, you will have a chance to observe and then reduce any compensations you might be making with your arms and notice how these adjustments affect how you are using your hips.

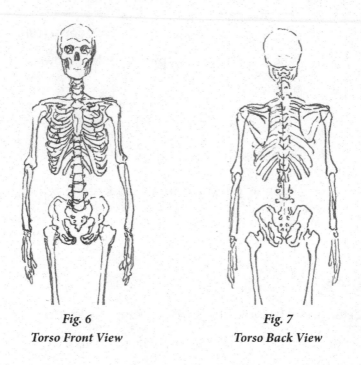

Fig. 6
Torso Front View

Fig. 7
Torso Back View

The following awareness building activity will help you under-stand and discover how your arms connect to your HNB and from there, influence your full body movement. It is important to consider your arms from both the front and back in order to develop your awareness of their volume. Remember to look at the accompanying video for more images and clarity.

Awareness Building
Arms

(Video #6: Arms)

As you observe the following in the lists below, notice the elegant design of the body, how if you happen to fall on your hands, the joints of your arms along with your rib cage act as shock absorbers protecting your heart and lungs (your vital organs). Take as much time as you need embodying each of these aspects of your arms from the back as from the front.

Refer to the drawing as you use your hands to explore the bones and connections mentioned below. Gaining this tactile sense will help you fill in the mental map of how your arms integrate into your overall structure.

Front View:

- Start in the middle of your torso at the top of your sternum. Feel how from both sides of the sternum, your clavicles (also known as collar bones) extend, reaching out on either side to connect to the bones of your arms.

- From there, feel how your shoulder joints are out to the sides of your body.

- Notice how the shoulder joint is actually mostly in the shoulder blade.

- Feel that there is space between the inside of your arms and the sides of your body.

Back View:

- Take your hands now to the back of your body and notice that your shoulder blades are quite high on your back.

- Consider whether the size of the shoulder blades matches your image of them.

- Notice how much distance there is between each shoulder blade and the spine.

- Use your hands and feel how the shoulder blades connect to your spine and ribs only by muscles and ligaments.

- With this awareness now, move your arms around and notice how easy and fluid the movements can be when you also allow the shoulder blades to move.

Legs

In a manner similar to the arms, the legs connect into the HNB and are critical in maintaining the biotensegral integrity. They participate in our grosser movements of locomotion and are, for most of us, our main vehicle for getting around. They do not operate alone, however, but are part of a whole-body motion.

The legs are our most immediate connection to the ground and how we use them directly affects our hips. When we allow the joints of our legs (hips, knees, ankles, feet) to move in a well-coordinated way, they become the unobstructed conduits for the GRF. When this happens, there may be a sensation of lightness, an ease of effort as if the torso is just floating along.

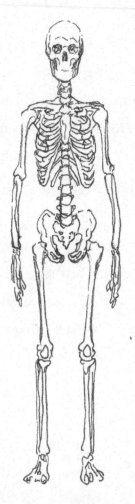
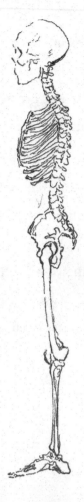

Fig. 8
Skeleton Front View

Fig. 9
Skeleton Side View

When you look at the skeletal structure from the front, you notice that the pelvis is wider than you might expect. A side view makes clear that the bones of the legs are in front of the spine. Awareness of these relationships allows for greater ease when sitting, standing, and walking.

The following Awareness Building Activity will help with developing an awareness of how your legs connect to your HNB and you can monitor the ease and fluidity with which you use them. It is also a chance to observe any compensations you may be making with your legs in relation to your hips. Consulting the accompanying video for more images and instructions will help refine this exploration.

Awareness Building
Legs

(Video #7: Legs)

It is important, however, to keep a sense of the back and front and volume of each of your legs as you work through the steps below.

Explore each step from a seated and a standing position. Notice what feels the same and what feels different about the two experiences. Like with the arm activity, using your hands will help you as you work to understand how your legs integrate into your overall structure. Again, take your time with each aspect listed below.

- Take a moment to sense the full dimensionality of your legs. Do this both seated and standing.

- Explore the motion of each of the leg joints. That means hips and ankles, as well as your knees. Notice how when you move from sitting to standing or standing to sitting as well as when you are walking, all of these joints are involved.

- Bring your attention now to your feet. Notice that your heels are behind and your toes are in front of your lower legs.

- Now that you have a fuller sense of your legs, notice how they are in front of your HNB. This may seem obvious when you are in a seated position. Once you come to a standing position, bring your attention to your tailbone and take note of how it and most of your pelvis are still behind your legs.

CHAPTER 3

The Hips

Whether or not you are anticipating hip surgery, refining your perception of your hips and their potential for mobility is a worthwhile endeavor. The instruction that follows prepares you for surgery and is a guide you can use during recovery. The essence of the work is how a conscious shift in thinking can create a greater sense of ease in the joints, the ripple effect of which is a sense of flow throughout the body.

The hips are a complex structure that function as the gateway between the legs and the rest of the body. How we perceive and experience this structure affects not only our equilibrium and stability but also how much effort we exert when walking, running, climbing stairs, etc. In order to access our best use, we must first develop a proper understanding of where the joints are within the hip system and how they function.

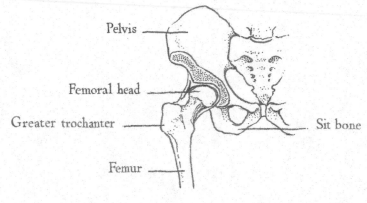

Fig. 10
Right Hip Joint

The hip joint can be mysterious and elusive. It is worth exploring in detail the various aspects of hip joint anatomy and how the joint relates to the rest of your pelvis.

It is common to think the bend in the hip joint occurs either at the side of the body at the greater trochanter or higher up at the top of the pelvic crest. Proper articulation occurs much closer to the midline of the body, in the ball and socket which you can see in the image above. Just becoming aware of this difference can unleash a profound sense of ease throughout your entire structure.

This bears repeating. Acquiring a more refined mental image of the hip joint and integrating that perception into your movement takes unnecessary pressure and stress off the rest of your body, allowing you to move more efficiently. The following Awareness Building Activities will help you discover your hip joints in relation to the rest of your body. You'll first look at the hip joint as part of your overall anatomy. From there, you will explore this information in motion. Consulting the accompanying videos for this second part can be extremely helpful.

Awareness Building
Hip Joint

Bring your awareness to the following aspects of your hip joint anatomy. Allow your awareness to expand as you sense the different parts of your structure. Developing a mental map of this anatomical arrangement is a prerequisite for changing your patterns of movement.

- The location of the hip joint is different from—and deeper than—the greater trochanter, the part of the femur you can feel on the outside of the leg.

- The hip joint is close to the body's midline.

- The hip joints are in the front half of your pelvis.

- The sit bones are below the hip joints.

- Your pubic bone is below and between the hip joints.

- The tailbone is behind the hip joints and slightly above the sit bones.

Movement Activity
Hip Joint Clarity

(Video #8: Hip Joint)

Below is a list of aspects of your hip joints. As you observe these aspects in the detailed image above, begin to sense them in your body. Remember how you used your hands to discover the clavicle leading to the arms and do the same here, letting your hands find the bony landmarks first and then the places where movement occurs.

Let yourself explore and discover. Be curious. Allow yourself to have a new experience, even if you think your current sense of your hips is sufficient.

- Use your hands to find the greater trochanters at the top of the outsides of your legs. You will feel them several inches below the rim of your pelvis.

- Keep your hands there while you tilt your torso forward, head going out over your knees. Notice the movement occurring with the fold at the top of your thighs.

- Come back to the vertical, still keeping your hands on your greater trochanters.

- Now, walk your fingers from the greater trochanters around the front of your hip folds towards your midline, stopping where you think your hip sockets are located based on the image above.

- Tilt forward again. Now rock on your sit bones while sensing the fold in your hip joints. This should help you feel that the hip joints are above the sit bones.

- Rock your torso back and forth slowly, focusing on just the movement of the hip joint. As you isolate this action, you can allow it to deepen into the socket and become more refined.

- Use the image above to help you think of your femurs (also known as the thigh bones) going back towards your hip sockets. Just having this thought can increase the fold in the joint.

- Pause now in this forward tilt and let go of any extra muscular tension. Next, bring your awareness to sense the full length of your HNB. Keeping this awareness along with a sense of ease in the hip joint, bring yourself back to an upright sitting posture.

Take a moment to integrate what you have just experienced. Allow yourself to embody this new sense of space within the structure of your hips and pelvis.

Continue to play with these Movement and Awareness Activities, letting yourself notice how your thoughts and movements affect one another. Take your time and feel free to study the images in these first three chapters as much as you need. Increasingly, you will sense how your hips fit into your overall structure and how you may be accommodating any interferences in your flow. The more you work with these concepts, continuing to refine your sensory experience, the more progress you will make. The subtlety of this exploration is, thankfully, endless. Stay curious.

CHAPTER 4

Cultivating New Movement Patterns – How We Can Change

Now that you have a mental map of where your hips fit into the overall structure of your body, you are ready to examine your habits of movement and the thoughts that precede them.

F. M. Alexander has given us a practical way to develop this awareness. It involves cultivating our sense of the intimate connection between our thoughts, posture, and movements. Becoming aware of our thoughts and the fact that we have the ability to decide how to move before we actually do so is the *means* to making different and better choices.

Alexander's process is fairly simple in theory. In practice, however, we encounter our long-standing, often unconscious perceptions and habits. Once there is an awareness that we can change, steps can be taken to consider what other options are available and how to consciously make better choices.

Four Key Elements:

STIMULUS – GAP – CHOICE – RESPONSE

The **STIMULUS** is any urge or thought to accomplish something. It can arise internally, like the desire for a cookie or the need to sit down. It can also come from external sources like a stoplight turning green or hearing someone call your name. Consider the examples below and whether they might be internal or external.

- Reaching for a pen.

- Putting your hands on your keyboard.

- Standing up from sitting.

- Shifting your weight to one foot.

- Taking a step.

- Stepping up on a curb.

- Swinging a tennis racket to hit an oncoming ball.

- Starting your backswing when the moment feels right to hit the golf ball.

If you found that some of the stimuli above could be either external or internal or both, you are on to something. Stimuli can come from multiple sources at once—doorbell ringing, child crying, and toast burning all at the same time. Even the most simple stimulus activates more stimuli, all unfolding in rapid succession.

A stoplight turning green, for example, is an external stimulus that initiates a sequence of internal stimuli. Before you respond to the green light, a lot has to take place. Awareness of this is the first step towards change.

GAP stands for **Give A Pause**. A pause is a moment of deliberate non-doing in which your awareness remains active. It is about taking a moment before taking action. In that moment, you have the opportunity to *not* do what you normally do and instead consciously *wait*. Yes, just wait. By waiting, you stop yourself from proceeding automatically. It is during the time of waiting where you find the space to inhibit your habit and invite the possibility of doing things differently.

The GAP is *the* pivotal moment. At once, fleeting and capable of expanding exponentially, it is an interlude before the response, a chance for myriad possibilities to arise.

From there, a process unfolds. It starts with dropping any physical or mental preparation that may have already occurred. This interlude is an opportunity to re-find your balance. It is a place of non-doing in which you are free to consider what **CHOICE** will lead you to a more efficient action.

CHOICE is what occurs in the GAP and allows you to develop what Alexander referred to as *conscious control*. How and what you choose becomes the basis for your next movement. Practicing this over time enables you to refine your awareness to the point that you can choose directions that will lead you to rebalance your system and find more ease.

Choice brings you out of automatic pilot and into an opportunity for change. It bears repeating: As you practice this, the process will become more familiar and the sensations will become increasingly subtle and nuanced.

Finally, we get to **RESPONSE,** the point at which you take action based on your new-found balance and flow. At first, the sensation and outcome may feel unfamiliar, even wrong. Don't panic. Stay with the process and get curious. This is where having an attitude of curiosity and non-judgment are essential. Keep exploring the sensory changes without labeling them good or bad. If everything felt the same, you would be just repeating your old habit.

Let's explore each step of this four-part process for change, using answering the phone as the activity.

Awareness Building
GAP Practice

STIMULUS

Your phone is ringing.

- Notice the moment you first hear the phone.

- Notice where your mind goes.

  - Who is calling?

  - Do you have time for a call?

  - Is this interrupting your other thoughts or activities?

GAP

- Pause.

- Take a moment to find your balance.

- Breathe.

CHOICE

- Notice any automatic movements, macro or micro, physical or mental, that you may have made or want to make in preparation for action.

- Let those go.

- Return to non-doing.

- Continue to wait in the pause.

- Notice what thoughts and urges are coming up.

- Let those go, and again, return to non-doing.

- Direct yourself to rebalance your system and structure. Do this by:

  - Sensing the ground underneath you.

  - Notice the GRF returning back up through your structure.

  - Allow your head to balance on your spine.

  - Maintain ease and fluidity in your joints.

  - Sense the space between the top of your head and the ceiling.

  - Sense the volume of your body.

  - Notice the space around your body in the room.

  - Inhale and feel your breath circulate throughout your body.

  - Allow visual images to come toward you.

  - Allow sounds to float through you.

RESPONSE - Move with Ease

- Pick up the phone.

- Greet the caller (if they are still there).

- Notice the difference in your response, physically and emotionally, when you have paused before answering

Movement Activity
GAP Applied to the Hips

The following activity directly applies the GAP process to the hips. Start from a seated situation.

STIMULUS

You want to stand up.

- Notice why you want to stand.

GAP

- Pause.

- Breathe in and breathe out.

CHOICE

- Bring your attention to your hip joints.

- Take a moment to release them and sense your weight on the supporting surface of your chair.

- Bring your awareness to your entire torso, sit bones to head.

- Breathe.

RESPONSE - Move with Ease

- Tilt your torso forward allowing the hips to bend at the joints.

- Continue bending the hips as much as needed in order to transfer your weight to your feet.

- Feel your feet on the ground.

- Allow your head to lead you up and out over your knees.

- Allow your body to unfold until you are standing upright.

CHAPTER 5

Start Where You are Now

Now that you are familiar with the concepts of *biotensegrity* and *unified field of awareness*, have started developing a more accurate body image, and are practicing the GAP process for change, you have the tools to develop what Alexander calls *reliable sensory appreciation*.

This chapter is an opportunity to develop a more embodied sense of these concepts. It will be a reality check, the next step in aligning your thinking with your physical experience. It will allow you to appreciate where you are with your current hip situation and understand possibilities for change and improvement.

As you go through the following steps, it is important to refrain from labeling yourself in any way or falling into a frame of mind that keeps you from a potential shift. Rather than thinking "That is just how it is" or "This will never change", ask yourself "How can I release that pattern?" or "What will it be like when that compensation is gone?"

This might sound too positive and even impossible at the moment. Don't despair. Even entertaining a thought or an image of the possibility that things can be different is enough to initiate change.

As your awareness increases and a sense of possibility emerges, there may come a moment when everything seems *wrong* or *bad*. It can at times feel disconcerting. This can be part of the process as awareness grows to include what has been occurring all along.

Again, don't despair, keep going. Taking the time to do this assessment will help you see what you will be focusing on and how much you can shift once you apply the GAP process.

The activity below has three parts. You will need a mirror, recent photos of yourself from the front, back, and side, and a current video of yourself standing and walking. The first part you will do on your own. Be honest and compassionate with yourself.

Awareness Building
Self-Observation

Start by viewing yourself from the front and side. Notice what general impressions emerge. You may need to take a moment to get past the initial feeling of surprise and "I'm too _____" phases of looking at yourself. Document these observations.

Next, watch yourself as you stand and walk. Notice what catches your eye and take note of these observations as well.

Taking this a step further, ask yourself the bulleted questions below and continue to note your answers.

Standing:

- Are your joints free and fluid or are you locking them?

- Is the musculature built-up in one area of your body more than another?

- Are you upright?

- Where is your head in relation to your pelvis?

- Where is your head in relation to your hips and feet?

- Is any part of your body—head, chest, pelvis—tilted to one side?

- Is one hip higher than the other?

- Is one hip more forward than the other?

Walking:

- What are your overall impressions?

- What is the first part of your body to move when you start to take a step?

- Are your steps equal in length?

- Where are your feet pointing?

- Is your head out ahead of your body?

- Are you tilted forward or back?

- Is your torso tilting to one side?

- Are your arms moving freely?

Now, for part two of the activity. Find someone who has your best interests in mind and a good eye for movement. Make sure this person is encouraging and non-judgmental. A kind voice and an easy tone will make it easier to hear what they are saying. Clear and specific feedback can be extremely helpful and inspiring.

Awareness Building
External Feedback

Have the observer look at your photos and videos. Then have them watch you as you move and ask them the same questions you asked yourself. Allow them to observe in silence. Make sure they are noting their answers.

- Notice if your movement changes because you know you are being observed.

- Listen to any feedback from your observer without needing to respond.

- Refrain from "fixing" anything.

- Mentally note what you sense your observer is seeing.

Now for part three.

Awareness Building
Comparing Feedback

With your observer, repeat the activity one more time. Discuss the similarities and differences you both noted.

- Get curious about any differences in your observations.

- Refrain from resolving to "fix" anything.

- Enjoy this exchange of information as yet another step in the process.

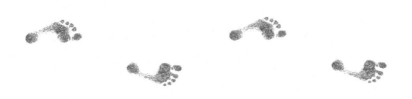

CHAPTER 6

Walking as Your Laboratory

Walking, our most basic mode of locomotion, is the ideal laboratory for continuing our exploration. It is an opportunity to deepen your awareness of the process that occurs between thoughts and actions. While this investigation is useful for anyone at any time, it is particularly relevant for those with hip concerns.

It is possible that developing this awareness can delay or even negate the need for surgery. When surgery is necessary, however, this training of the mind-body connection is critical. If you are looking at potential surgery, you do not need to wait for your hip to be fixed. You can begin retraining yourself now. When you do this, not only are you setting yourself up for an easier surgery, you are also preparing for a faster and more successful recovery.

So, walking. As you may have guessed, there is much to consider as you put one foot in front of the other. Using the GAP process of awareness, we will break the motion down into the sequence of components essential for a fluid gait.

As you play with the activity below, bringing your focus to the local parts of your body (hips, knees, ankles), be sure to continuously return your awareness to your whole self (the distance from your head to your feet and your full dimensionality). Too much focus on a local body part can disrupt the whole body's coordination and cause unnecessary movement patterns. Progress occurs more quickly when you constantly consider the local in relationship to the whole. As you continue exploring, you discover new sensations and open yourself to new ways of thinking.

Movement Activity
Walking Observation

(Video #9: Walkng)

In the previous chapter's activity, you and your partner observed yourself standing and walking in order to note your overall posture and alignment. In this activity, you will focus on your coordination while walking.

As you did before, watch yourself in a mirror and/or video as you walk.

- See what you notice.

- Note whether the movements you observe match what you think you are doing.

- Notice where you may be compensating and where a sense of ease may be emerging.

Continue observing as you ask yourself the following questions:

- What does it take to move my body weight forward?

- How much force and muscular effort do I use to move forward?

- How is my torso participating as I walk?

- What thoughts am I having?

- Am I pulling myself along?

- Am I pushing from the back foot?

- Am I falling forward onto the front leg?

- Am I pushing my hip forward before my leg moves?

- Do I grab the floor with my feet?

Considering these questions demands subtle attention. Notice where your thoughts go as you walk.

Taking this activity a step further, consider what happens when you think of walking as:

- A full-body activity.

- Requiring very little effort.

- A chance to sense the rebound from the earth's gravitational pull.

- A means of moving horizontally along the earth's surface.

- As a gliding motion, fluid and free.

The following are specific ideas and activities that will help you to find greater ease in walking.

Awareness Building
Supporting and Gesturing Legs

The supporting leg is the one bearing your weight. The non-weight-bearing leg is your gesturing leg.

Take a moment to stand in place and transfer your weight from side to side, noting how each leg goes from supporting to gesturing and back to supporting. Walk in place and note how much time you spend on one leg or the other and how little time you are on both legs at once.

Now, slow this movement down even further and bring your attention to the leg that is currently supporting. Notice the following:

- The overall length of the *supporting* leg.

- The length of this leg as an extension of the length (head to foot) of your entire structure.

- The pliability of the leg joints (hips, knees, and ankles) and how that influences the body's dynamic balance.

- Your foot spreading out on the floor.

Now, bring your attention to the *gesturing* leg. While it is not taking any weight and has a chance to recuperate, notice the following:

- The overall length of the *gesturing* leg, even while it is folding and extending.

- Maintaining your awareness of length (from head to foot) of your *supporting* leg while the *gesturing* leg moves.

- How the hip, knee and ankle all participate as the *gesturing* leg moves.

- The ease in all your leg joints as the *gesturing* leg swings through from back to front.

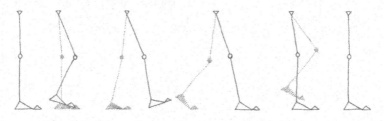

Fig. 11
Walking Chunks

Chunking-Up Walking

This section organizes walking into accessible actions, what we will refer to as "chunks". A GAP is inserted between each action or chunk (refer back to Chapter 4 for the GAP discussion) as an opportunity to think through directions before moving on to the next action or chunk.

Notice in Fig. 11 above that the majority of each step is spent balancing on one leg and time spent on two legs at once is only about one-third of the total stride. At this most fundamental level, walking is the repetitive action of balancing on one leg, then the other, over and over again.

Breaking the sequence down into small units allows enough time for the joints involved to function as best as they can. This slowed-down process also allows you the time and space to experience how gravity can support and vitalize your entire structure. These movements may feel artificial at first, like you are moving in slow motion. That is normal. Once you return to walking at your normal pace, the exercise of breaking down the movement into pieces will stay with you and you'll feel the individual chunks beginning to flow together.

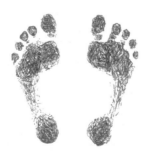

Fig. 12
Standing on Two Feet

Standing on Two Feet

Standing on both feet at once for a moment provides an opportunity to re-establish a sense of dimensionality, volume, and balance. This seemingly simple exercise is a practice in and of itself. For those with hip concerns, it is a critical part of pre- and post-surgery work. Using a deliberate pause in order to recalibrate is the first step in effectively moving forward.

Movement Activity
Standing on Two Feet

Start by standing on two feet and consciously pendulating from side to side, then from front to back. As you do this, notice your weight moving through your body, into the ground and through different parts of your feet. Also bring your attention back to your full dimensionality and volume. Notice how this simple movement connects you with your natural verticality and the rebound from gravity.

Observing yourself in a mirror may help you to more fully engage with this practice.

To take this a bit further, as you continue standing on two feet:

- Sense both feet on the floor.

- Allow your feet to spread out.

- Starting with ankles and working all the way up to the jaw and top of the spine, let your whole structure be free and fluid.

- From there, begin shifting your body weight from side to side.

- Continue to feel this rocking motion as you incrementally diminish it until your weight is evenly distributed on both feet.

- Repeat this swaying action, this time from front to back, from the balls of your feet to the back of your heels.

- As before, feel this rocking motion as you incrementally diminish it until your weight is evenly distributed on both feet.

- As you stop rocking and come into your verticality, you may sense that you no longer have to *hold* yourself up. This organization of your structure offers the most direct route for sensing gravity and the GRF as it runs through you.

Now we are going to integrate this awareness into the action of walking, applying what we have just discovered while on two feet to the motion of moving from one foot to the other. We will be breaking the act of walking into seven chunks in order that you can feel what it is like to maintain the sense of connectivity to gravity and the GRF throughout the process. Again, working with the video will be an important support.

Movement Activity
Walking

(Video #9: Walking)

By dividing the act of walking into seven chunks and inserting a GAP between each chunk, you have the opportunity to re-adjust as you go. Each GAP guides you deeper into a better balance. Consistently reinitiating these directions throughout the act of walking reinforces your best use as you go. Depending on the state of your hip health, you may want to have a mobility aid or wall nearby to help you balance during the GAPs.

Chunk #1 Prepare to walk.

- Sense both feet on the floor.

- Distribute your weight as evenly as possible between your footprints.

- Bring your awareness to releasing all of your joints, letting your whole structure be fluid and free.

- Now, add an awareness of your hips to the whole and allow your weight to flow through your hips into the ground.

Keep your breath flowing and your joints easy, while sensing the distance from your head to your feet and from your feet to your head. **GAP** Reset your balance.

- Reinitiate a sense of the gravitational pull and the simultaneous rebound up through your entire system.

- Notice your length, width, depth, and full dimensionality.

- Allow your breath to move through you.

- Sense the space inside your body and around you.

Chunk #2 Think about taking a step forward onto your right foot.

- Do not take that step.

- Stand on both feet.

- Notice what your body started to do.

- Notice if you are preparing or anticipating in any way.

GAP Reset your balance.

- Reinitiate a sense of the gravitational pull and the simultaneous rebound up through your entire system.

- Notice your length, width, depth, and full dimensionality.

- Allow your breath to move through you.

- Sense the space in your body and around you.

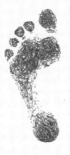

Fig. 13

Chunk #3 Shift to the left leg.

- Shift your weight onto your left foot keeping your entire right foot lightly contacting the floor (see Fig. 13).

- Let your weight fall through the midline of your foot near the back of the inner arch.

GAP Reset your balance.

- From where you are, reinitiate a sense of the gravitational pull and the simultaneous rebound up through your entire system.

- Notice your length, width, depth, and full dimensionality.

- Allow your breath to move through you.

- Sense the space in your body and around you.

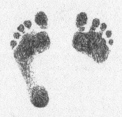

Fig. 14

Chunk #4 Right knee moves forward.

- Bring the right knee forward from the back of your knee.

- Release the ankle.

- Allow the heel to come off of the floor.

- The metatarsals and toes of the right foot are touching the floor without bearing any weight (see Fig. 14).

- Let your weight fall through the midline of your foot near the back of the inner arch.

- Notice the length from your right knee to your right hip.

GAP Reset your balance.

- From where you are, reinitiate a sense of the gravitational pull and the simultaneous rebound up through your entire system.

- Notice your length, width, depth, and full dimensionality.

- Allow your breath to move through you.

- Sense the space in your body and around you.

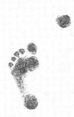

Fig. 15

Chunk #5 Right heel touches the floor in front of you.

- Keep your weight completely on your left foot, letting your weight fall through the midline near the back of the inner arch.

- Meanwhile, extend your right leg forward a short distance, letting only the heel touch the floor in front of you (see Fig. 15).

- Do not take any weight on the heel of this gesturing right leg yet.

- In this suspended state with your weight still only on your left foot, sense the GRF coming up through both the supporting left leg and the heel of the gesturing right leg, through your body, and out the top of your head.

GAP Reset your balance.

- From where you are, reinitiate a sense of the gravitational pull and the simultaneous rebound up through your entire system.

- Notice your length, width, depth, and full dimensionality.

- Allow your breath to move through you.

- Sense the space in your body and around you.

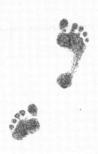

Fig. 16

Chunk #6 Shift your weight over the front right foot.

- Keeping your body long by thinking of your length from the tailbone to the top of your spine, shift your center of gravity forward by taking your head over your right foot.

- As you shift forward, allow the left knee and the left big toe to bend, leaving only your left metatarsal on the floor (see Fig. 16).

- Notice your left big toe helping you balance without bearing weight.

GAP Reset your balance.

- From here, reinitiate a sense of the gravitational pull and the simultaneous rebound up through your entire system.

- Notice your length, width, depth, and full dimensionality.

- Allow your breath to move through you.

- Sense the space in your body and around you.

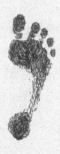

Fig. 17

Chunk #7 Swing the left leg through.

- Continue standing on your right leg completely (see Fig. 17).

- Left leg comes forward, bending from the back of the knee.

- Let the left leg swing through, releasing the left ankle.

- Extend the left leg a short distance forward towards the floor.

- Let the left heel contact the floor in front of you.

GAP Reset your balance.

- From here, reinitiate a sense of the gravitational pull and the simultaneous rebound up through your entire system.

- Notice your length, width, depth, and full dimensionality.

- Allow your breath to move through you.

- Sense the space in your body and around you.

Movement Activity
GAP IN MOTION

Now it is time to put it all together, first slowly, then at your normal pace. Take your time and stay curious as you take this new knowledge and coordination into your daily life.

Deliberate Slow Walking:

- Move through the sequence of chunks and GAPs, sensing your forward motion.

- Take time to register each chunk.

- Remember the GAPs.

- Register which leg is supporting and which is gesturing.

- Note as the legs transition from supporting to gesturing and vice versa.

- Notice yourself balancing on one leg most of the time.

Walking at Your Normal Pace:

- Notice how your body responds as you pick up your pace.

- Bring your thoughts back to the chunking process.

- Continue to insert the GAPs.

- Any time you come to a stop and find yourself back on two feet, use this pause to reinitiate your directions.

- If you find yourself returning to previous habits or going on autopilot, let yourself pause. Take a moment to remember your directions, then start again.

- Go slowly at first, inserting the GAPs, and as you feel ready, pick up the pace.

CHAPTER 7

Deepen, Refine &
Expand Your Awareness

So far, we have looked at elements of the body and the concept
of *unified field of awareness*. But there is more. What follows
involves more nuanced or refined elements of our function and
perception. Each element could become its own extended exploration. For our purposes, however, an overview will deepen our
inquiry into hip health.

As you read on, continue exploring with the same intention
and attention you have applied previously. Be curious, patient,
and playful.

Sensory Awareness

Sight, sound, taste, touch, smell. We receive all our information
through our senses. They are our means of perceiving the world
and we each have our own preferred senses. For example, one
person might tune first into all the sounds around them, while

someone else might be most sensitive to color, or movement, or smell. We assume everyone else is perceiving the world as we are. In actuality, we each have a unique sensory lens.

Identifying and beginning to work with your sensory preferences can be life changing. Understanding how you best take in information can open the world up to you in a way you have not experienced before. When it comes to working with hip issues, change for some might come through seeing yourself moving differently, while others may need to feel or hear that change. When you tune into your dominant sense and let it guide you, you may find change happening effortlessly and the way forward becoming quite clear.

Awareness Building
Senses

The list below calls on a variety of senses. Some will feel more comfortable and more accessible to you than others. Noticing this difference, it is part of identifying your preferences. Let the preferred sense be your way into those that feel less familiar. By doing so, you will expand your capacity for change.

Clear your mind of any preconceived notions as you take yourself through the list below. Be open to possibility and be honest about what feels good and what feels foreign. There is no right or wrong. Whatever you experience is valuable information.

- Notice any sounds around you and even within you.

- Extend that noticing to include sounds in the expanded environment.

- Note the temperature of the air around you.

- Register any light coming towards you.

- See any shadows in the space.

- Take in the colors of your environment.

- Bring your attention to the shapes of items or objects around you.

- Feel the air against your skin.

- Notice any odors or scents.

- Feel the texture of your clothes against your skin.

- Note any tastes you have in your mouth.

Having gone through this list once noticing your preferences, go through it again. This time, start with your preferred sense, then add in one or more of your less dominant senses. For example, if sight is your main mode of taking in information, focus on something in your environment. As you are seeing, layer in your ability to also hear. You can practice this endlessly, in myriad variations. There is no limit to this exploration.

Eye Focus

While all the senses affect our balance and function, the eyes demand special attention. In fact, sight has become the dominant sense for most of us in today's world. Our eyes lead us through our day—where they go, we follow. Think about it: when we look at the ground, we often pull our head down and even a bit forward. When we raise our gaze back up to eye-level, however, our body returns to a more upright stance.

The next step in becoming more aware of how our eyes affect our movement and function is to remember that they are basically receptors. In the same way that looking down may pull us forward, using our eyes to grab at objects in our environment can also pull us too far forward. Both of these habits can take us off our best balance.

The following Movement Activity is a useful practice for keeping the focus flexible and responsive to whatever comes along.

Movement Activity
Eye Focus

Explore this list first while you are seated. Go through it again while you are in motion. Notice where you are looking and how that affects your balance and posture.

- Start by softening your eye muscles.

- Allow your eyes to rest in the eye sockets.

- Let the light come towards you.

- Maintaining this easy focus, notice what is immediately in front of you.

- Gently expand this focus to include the ground 2-3 feet around you.

- Continue to extend your gaze to encompass a still larger area.

- Now bring your awareness to maintaining a sense of both the near space and the larger area.

- Continue to breathe.

- Maintaining this awareness, layer in your peripheral vision.

- Breathe.

- See one specific object, while maintaining your sense of near, far, and peripheral.

- Release your attention on that object and return to allowing your eyes to relax and receive.

- Breathe.

As you work with your eye focus and attend to the subtleties of your movements, you will start to sense how your overall balance is affected. When it comes to your hips, discovering the role your eyes play in managing your balance is a big step. Pay particular attention to what happens to your hips when you look to one side or the other. Looking straight ahead, avoiding any twisting if you are having hip issues, may be a way to stay pain-free.

Breathing

You may have noticed that breathing is a recurring step in the previous activity. That is because it plays a critical role in finding our best balance and posture. While breathing, for most of us, happens automatically, bringing a conscious awareness to it can maximize its functioning.

We all want our breathing to be easy and free. There is more to it, though. Our breath when allowed its full potential, supports our dimensionality and helps us tune into an innate flow.

Use the next Movement Activity to explore your breathing process. If at any time you feel odd or lightheaded, pause. When you feel better, start again—but this time more slowly.

Movement Activity
Breathing

Take a moment to slow your inhale-exhale. As you do so, take yourself through the following checklist. Allow your breath to move easily, fully, freely, without trying to "do" anything.

- Close your lips and let the air flow in and out through your nose.

- Notice how the air can move without any muscular pushing or pulling.

- Let the inhale expand your ribs gently to the sides

- Let the exhale soften the ribs as you breathe out.

- Sense the inhale supporting the length of your body from the top of your head to your pelvic floor.

- Even though it is not the main movement, notice the subtle movement of your abdomen.

- Let your shoulders be easy and wide.

- Let your jaw be easy.

- Relax your tongue.

- Soften your eyes.

- Let your head balance on your spine.

Cross-Patterning

The right-left coordination we develop when learning to crawl as babies is known as cross-patterning. This action activates supportive connections throughout the body and enables us to evolve the capacity to bend, extend, twist, and spiral in multiple dimensions. It is what allows us to maintain our balance even though we may be turning to the right or to the left.

Cross-patterning is an essential part of walking. When our bodies are free and easy, cross-patterning occurs naturally and automatically as a means of stabilizing our bodies.

Cross-patterning can be disrupted when our movement becomes restricted. This, of course, is readily apparent for those of us with hip issues. We adjust our movements as a way of minimizing pain and allowing our continued mobility. The recognition of these adjustments, or compensations, is important in addressing any shifts in our cross-patterning that may be compromising our stability.

The Movement Activity that follows will activate your cross-patterning and help sort out issues of imbalance.

Movement Activity
Cross-Patterning

In preparation for this activity, stand on both feet with your arms at your sides. Allow your body to adjust ever so slightly until you feel your weight evenly distributed.

- Shift your weight to the right foot.

- Bring your left knee up toward your midline. Touch your left knee with your right hand. Allow your whole body to respond to your hand meeting your knee.

- Return to standing on both feet with your arms at your sides.

- Shift your weight to your left foot.

- Bring your right knee up toward your midline. Touch your right knee with your left hand. Allow your whole body to respond to this movement.

- Return to standing on both feet with your arms at your sides.

- Repeat this several times.

- When you are finished, stop and stand on both feet.

- Notice any difference in how you feel your weight is distributed.

- Now, walk forward noticing if you sense any change in your balance.

- As you walk, allow your arms to swing in opposition to your legs. When your left foot takes your weight, your right arm is also forward. As your right foot then comes forward, so does your left arm.

- Stop. Stand once again on both feet. Take a moment to stand in stillness and notice your balance.

Spatial Awareness

When you are experiencing your best balance, your awareness is able to expand beyond your own body to include the space around you. This expanded awareness is also a crucial part of maintaining balance.

Engaging with this *global* awareness then becomes a source of support. And, movement is no longer a matter of muscular *doing* but a release into spatial *allowing*.

In Chapter 1, we spoke about spatial thinking as it relates to overall body image, dimensionality, and biotensegrity. We want now to expand this concept to include the space immediately around us. From there, we can extend this concept to include a bigger and bigger space until we eventually even include outer space.

Awareness Building
Spatial Awareness

Use the list below to explore the continuum of space, moving from inside to outside and then all around and beyond your body. You are training your mind to perceive *locally* and *globally,* simultaneously.

- Reconnect with the space inside your body. Sense your length, width, depth, and volume.

- Expand that awareness into the space just beyond your body's boundaries.

- Extend that bigger awareness now to include the entire room.

- Now let your awareness include the space beyond the room. This continued opening has no limits as it moves outside any structures into the great outdoors.

Notice what emerges as you maintain this expanded spatial awareness. You can continue expanding your field of awareness on into forever. The only requirement is that you simultaneously maintain a sense of your own body. It is a rewarding skill to cultivate and can bring you to a whole new state of being.

Working with Your Pain

When we are in pain, we often defer to the familiar. We fall back on what we know, even if these habits are what caused the pain in the first place. It is difficult in these moments with pain dominating our awareness to feel capable of doing things differently.

We do have a choice, however. When we train ourselves to pause (even when it feels impossible) and shift our focus, we can begin to work *with* the pain, no longer spending our energy on trying to stop it. In this way, our pain becomes yet another tool for discovering alternate ways of moving and thinking.

Awareness Building
Working with Your Pain

Start by acknowledging and even accepting the pain. Surely, this seems counterintuitive but even a moment's worth of sitting with your pain rather than trying to stop it is enough to shift things.

- Notice where the pain is in your body.

- Allow your awareness of the pain to expand to adjacent parts of your body.

- If you haven't already, allow your entire limb or body part to come into your awareness.

- Let your attention continue to spread, including more and more of your body.

- Now, let that awareness extend out into the space around you.

Take a moment to notice how this process of integrating the pain into the whole allows it to dissipate, disperse, even dissolve.

Now, do this again, this time sensing the whole from a place that feels good.

- Find a place in your body that feels calm.

- Allow this good feeling to expand.

- If you haven't already, let the pleasant sensation spread to the entire limb or part of your body.

- Continue to let this sense of ease spread until it includes your entire body.

- Spend a little extra time with those parts of the body that are in pain. It is possible to experience both simultaneously. So don't give up. Let the pleasant sensation absorb the pain.

CHAPTER 8

Thinking and Moving in Action

We have spent the last chapters developing awareness. It is time to apply this awareness to simple motions we do on a daily basis. This is possible through the use of strategies that are fundamental to improving balance and managing pain. This chapter also includes a handful of activities to keep yourself mobile.

Keep Moving

We cannot underestimate the importance of continuing to move. Not only do breathing, circulation and heart health benefit from movement, our joint mobility is directly affected by whether or not we keep moving.

Movement does not need to be rigorous or even aerobic. There is no need to stress or strain. What is important is that we keep moving, and the more we move, the better. This will differ depending on each person's hip status—that means range of motion and level of pain. No matter where you are with your hip health, the goal is to maintain and if possible, improve upon your current condition and coordination.

Mobility Aids

Mobility aids can help you minimize compensations, feel more stable, and possibly avoid developing habits you will need to undo after surgery. Allowing yourself to use a mobility aid may be a big step, psychologically. Keep in mind, it is likely just temporary and more importantly, it can prevent your condition from worsening while allowing you to move with as much balance and ease as possible.

If you find yourself leaning on furniture as you move around your house or making choices about not going out, consider how a cane could allow you to be more mobile. It is worth reassessing your need to appear "normal," and self-sufficient. Putting aside these concerns to use a cane or walker will allow you to keep moving and even help improve your posture.

Specific instructions for how best to work with mobility aids can be found in Appendix 1. Take the time to read through it and know that the best time to experiment with mobility aids is pre-surgery. If you are already using a cane or walker, Appendix 1 gives you tips on how to refine your use in order to maintain your best balance.

Helpful Movement Activities

Here is a series of ten activities that can help you to keep moving. They are simple movements with which you can have fun experimenting. If any of them feel uncomfortable, you can modify them by using a wall or chair for support. You can also not do them. These activities will provide you with a system for cultivating and practicing whole body coordination that will support the movement of your hips.

Work slowly, consciously, and at your own pace. Observe how the movements affect your breathing and mobility. Take breaks so both your body and mind have time to integrate any changes and discoveries. The shifts may be subtle but they accumulate to create significant change. Stay curious and enjoy the process!

Movement Activity
Small Movements

(Video #10: Small Movements)

This activity is very subtle yet powerful. You will see that the smallest movements reverberate throughout your system. A simple movement of the eyes can be felt in your hips. Developing an awareness of this chain reaction can help you to unlock some blocking of movement that may be occurring due to pain or a physical impingement.

Once you recognize the potential in your spine for movement, you can begin to work towards a new sense of mobility. These subtle movements work to then redistribute the tone in your torso and legs, helping you reconnect with the ground and GRF.

These activities can be done sitting, standing or lying down.

- Look forward.

- Let only your eyes look down toward your knees.

- Allow your head to follow your eyes.

- Notice that your pelvis and hips can respond.

- Raise your eyes to once again look forward.

- Let your head and body respond.

- Notice that your pelvis adjusts.

- Let your eyes look either to the left or right.

- Notice how your whole head, neck and back (including your pelvis and hips) respond to this smallest movement of your eyes.

- Look in the other direction, allowing your whole torso and hips to respond.

- Now come back to looking forward and sense the relationship of your head and whole torso.

Movement Activity
Moving Your Torso from Both Ends

(Video #11: Moving the Torso from Both Ends)

This next activity takes the subtle movement you have just done and makes it larger. Moving the torso now from both ends will help you further clarify your sense of the distance between the top of the head and the sit bones. This increased sense of connection also offers insight into how moving the hips affects and is affected by movement in other parts of the body.

This activity, too, can be done:

- On your hands and knees.

- Standing with your hands on the back of a chair or on a countertop.

- Standing with your hands against a wall.

- With your hands contacting the floor, chair or wall, move your head in any direction that feels good and allow your entire torso, including your hips, to respond.

- With your hands still in place, move your chest in any direction that feels good and allow your entire torso, including your head and hips, to respond.

- Come back to center.

- Hands still contacting your surface of choice, move your entire torso, head, and hips around in whatever way feels good.

- Return to center, noticing what you notice.

Movement Activity
Rolling Down, Rolling Up

(Video #12: Rolling Down, Rolling Up)

This next activity works along the midline using sequential and simultaneous movement in order to access more spatial clarity.

This activity is done while seated.

- Start by looking straight ahead with your hands on your thighs, keeping your torso vertical.

- Let your eyes see your knees. Moving from the top of your spine, slowly let your head follow.

- Letting your head lead, continue curling forward, allow your pelvis to respond.

- Without engaging your abdominal muscles, breathe out as you curl forward, going only as far as is comfortable.

- Remember your hands are on your thighs and as you curl forward, you can let your elbows go out to your sides.

- When you feel ready, breathe in, uncurling your torso and return to vertical.

Movement Activity
Roll Down with Torso Extension

(Video #13: Roll Down with Torso Extension)

This next activity also works along the midline to further integrate the coordination of head, neck, and back. Move slowly and only go as far as you are comfortable. Please, remember to watch the video.

This activity is also done while seated.

- Start by looking straight ahead with your hands on your thighs, keeping your torso vertical.

- Let your eyes see your knees. Moving from the top of your spine, slowly let your head follow.

- Letting your head lead, continue curling forward, allow your pelvis to respond.

- Without engaging your abdominal muscles, breathe out as you curl forward, going only as far as is comfortable.

- Taking this movement a step further, let your eyes look forward along the floor in front of you and let your head and torso follow, extending out over your thighs.

- This may feel awkward, but from this position, allow yourself to feel the length from the top of your head to your sit bones.

- Pause and breathe.

- Now let your eyes continue to see the floor, moving the focus all the way to the wall in front of you. Allow the torso to continue extending as the head lifts in sync with the eyes' sight line.

- Continue this movement until your torso is once again vertical.

- Let your eyes once again look forward and your head rebalance on the top of your spine.

- Notice if you are experiencing a greater sense of support and length through your head, neck, and back. This is the GRF finding a clearer path.

Movement Activity
Seated Spirals

(Video #14. Seated Spirals)

Seated spirals are yet another way of integrating the head, neck, and back.

This activity is done while seated.

- Start with your torso vertical. Look straight ahead and place your hands on your thighs.

- Take a moment to sense the full length of your head, neck, and back.

- Let your eyes lead as you slowly look to the right, letting your head and whole torso follow.

- Breathe out as you go and move only as far as is comfortable.

- Starting with your pelvis, reverse the sequence and breathe in as you return to face forward.

- Do this movement on the left side.

- Repeat this activity on both sides several times. Notice yourself moving more easily and farther each time, without any pushing or pulling.

Movement Activity
Re-establishing Your Balance

(Video #15: Re-establishing Your Balance)

Taking a moment to stand and re-establish your balance will allow you to appreciate the significance of the subtle movements of the previous activities. It is also a chance to integrate this more nuanced awareness into your increasingly refined sense of balance.

This activity is done standing, either

- With your arms at your sides.

- With your hands on the back of a chair or on a countertop.

- With your hands against a wall.

  - From the standing position that works best for you, allow your hips, knees, and ankles to be easy and pliable.

  - Notice your weight being supported evenly through both legs as much as possible.

  - Allow your spine to have its natural curves. (See Fig. 9, for a quick review).

- Allow your head to balance on your spine.

- Sense the weight of your body as it moves through your legs and feet into the floor and rebounds up through your body.

- Gradually diminish any arm support.

- Once again, sense the GRF as you find your best balance.

Movement Activity
Wall Push-ups

(Video #16: Wall Push-ups)

Wall push-ups are unique in their ability to help you find the full length of your body, from the top of your head straight out through your heels. This sense of length further refines your balance.

This activity is done standing facing a wall, at almost an arm's length distance.

- Find your balance on two feet.

- Place your palms on the wall at shoulder height, maintaining your verticality. Your hands should be just wider than your shoulders with elbows toward the floor and fingertips toward the ceiling.

- Bring your awareness to the length of your body, from your feet to the top of your head.

- Now, let your weight go into your hands and allow the length of your body to tilt toward the wall, subtly shifting off the vertical.

- Pause for a moment in this slight slant and sense your full length.

- From this new sense of length, push away from the wall, your body moving a whole, until you are again vertical and balanced.

- Remember to find your best balance on two feet before removing your hands from the wall.

- Repeat the exercise.

- Exhale as you lean toward the wall. While slanted, inhale into your length. Exhale again, as you push back to the vertical.

- Take this activity deeper by moving your feet farther away from the wall.

- Notice the connection from your hands to your feet and feet to your hands during this activity.

Movement Activity
Walking in Place

(Video #17: Walking in Place)

Walking in place helps you focus on and refine the movement of your legs without having to negotiate movement through space. This may seem familiar, as we broke down the walking sequence in Chapter 6. It is useful in this context as a good way to practice the coordination and refinement of your movement from one leg to the other.

This activity can be done:

- Standing without any support from your arms.

- Using one or both arms to stabilize yourself on the wall or back of a chair.

- Using one of your mobility aids.

- Shift your weight completely to one leg.

- Balance on that leg for support.

- The foot of your gesturing leg is still contacting the floor, even though it is taking no weight.

- Sense the length of the supporting side from foot to head.

- If you are contacting a support, use your hands to direct your body toward the vertical. It may feel like you are gently pushing away from your hands. This is the direction you want, rather than leaning into them.

- Allow the knee of the gesturing leg to come forward so that the foot of that leg is barely off the floor.

- Replace that foot on the floor.

- Balance equally on both legs.

- Repeat on the other side.

- Continue to walk in place like this. Take time to deliberately shift your weight from one side to the other.

Movement Activity
Sit to Stand – Stand to Sit

(Video #18: Sit to Stand – Stand to Sit)

Moving from sitting to standing and vice versa is an action most of us do many times a day without thinking. Bringing this action into deliberate focus will help make the motion more fluid and less effortful.

Start this activity while seated.

- Find your best seated vertical balance. Sense your sit bones on the chair, knees in front of your hip joints, and feet flat on the floor.

- Tilt forward with your head leading, allowing your pelvis to respond, rocking forward on your sit bones.

- Continue following your head out over your knees on about a 45° angle.

- Keep going until your head leads your body off your pelvic support and your body weight goes into the floor through your feet.

- Come to standing by directing your head up away from your feet, allowing your whole body to lengthen.

Continue this activity by returning to sitting.

- Allow your leg joints (hips, knees, ankles) to soften in preparation for movement.

- Stay balanced over your feet by continuing to bend at the hips, knees, and ankles while allowing your lengthened torso to tilt forward at about 45°.

- Continue folding until your pelvis lands on the chair.

- Allow your torso to return to vertical by taking your head back over your pelvis.

- Once again, find your best balance by letting go of any extra effort.

Movement Activity
Balancing on One Leg

(Video #19: Balancing on One Leg)

Again, as we learned in Chapter 6, each time we take a step, we are for a moment balancing on one leg. Isolating this one action serves to refine our overall balance and stability.

The activity is done standing. It can be done:

- Without any support from your arms.

- Using one or both arms to stabilize yourself on the wall or back of a chair.

- Using one of your mobility aids.

- Shifting your weight to one leg.

  - Bring the gesturing leg forward in front of you by bending your knee forward.

  - Focus on your length from foot to head on the supporting side.

  - Allow the supporting foot to spread out and feel the length from heel to toe.

  - Gradually diminish any support you may be getting from your arms.

- As you balance, use at least one arm to move around, challenging your stability.

- Remember to keep your joints pliable so you are able to rebalance with ease.

- Practice this balancing on the other leg.

- Challenge yourself by increasing the time you spend balancing on each leg.

Lie Down

You may also benefit from practicing the Lie Downs in Appendix II. Lie Downs help you integrate your new habits. The Balance Arts Center has a 10-minute audio download of a Lie Down available in multiple languages. To access, please visit: www.balanceartscenter.com/lie-down.

CHAPTER 9

Navigating Hip Surgery

The ideas and principles presented so far in this book allow you to cultivate best movement and postural habits. They provide an overarching attitude and approach that you can refer to as you interface with the world around you. For our purposes here, we use these ideas to now look at how best to approach the experience of hip surgery.

Note: It is important to keep in mind that wherever you are in your hip health journey, you can always dip back into pretty much anywhere in the previous chapters to work on any of the movement activities. Each time you revisit an activity, you benefit from fuller embodiment and integration.

The goal all along has involved expanding your awareness as a way of refining your ability to change. This does not stop with the prospect of surgery. In fact, to look at surgery as an opportunity to develop your awareness and supportive habits further can change your experience completely.

Adapt an attitude of exploration and continued learning. Set as your goal an overall sense of balance and ease. And keep your eye on your long-term wellness. Rather than limping or hitching up your hip to find relief from the pain, dare to use a cane or walker, knowing that such a mobility device will help with maintaining your best balance in both the immediate moment and long term.

If your hip health develops to the point where you have decided to go forward with surgery, there are many things to consider. While you will have your own unique set of medical and social circumstances, a basic checklist can be found in Appendix VI. The more details you handle prior to surgery, the freer you will be to more fully engage in the healing process.

If you have read this far into the book and your injury or hip surgery happened several years ago, you have no doubt already understood the value of the work presented here. It is never too late to resume your recovery.

When to Have Surgery

Most people wait too long. If you notice compensations in your movement, pain becoming more constant, activities you are avoiding to protect your hip, or an excess of mental energy spent managing your situation, it might be time to consult a doctor.

It is important to keep in mind that consulting a surgeon does not mean agreeing to surgery. Think of your visit as a fact-finding mission. Gathering several professional opinions regarding your particular case and the treatment options will enable you to make an informed decision.

Pre-surgery

Once you have chosen a surgeon, and together, you all have decided the time is right to move forward with surgery, you still may have to wait for a surgery date. This can be a good thing as it will give you time to prepare so that all can go as smoothly as possible.

In addition to all the logistical preparations, you can use this pre-surgery period as an opportunity to pay particular attention to your thinking and moving. The more intentional you can be about this part of your preparation, the faster and more fully you will recover.

You can start by reviewing the beginning chapters of this book to refresh how you think about your movement. Re-explore the exercises and notice how repeating an activity produces a new experience, as your awareness becomes further integrated. Resetting your attitude and approach to movement will release habits developed due to structural restrictions your hips have created.

All surgery comes with its fair share of fear and anxiety. Rather than pushing these feelings away, it can be helpful to acknowledge them and identify techniques for addressing them. If you are not already doing so, it might be a good time to start a mindfulness practice such as meditation as a complement to the movement work you have been doing.

Surgery

The best way to navigate the actual surgical process is to surrender to the system and processes of the doctors and facilities that are caring for you. You have done your research and can trust that the team you've chosen knows what they are doing.

While this may be a new experience for you, the procedures are meant to produce the best outcomes. Each individual on your surgery team has their own responsibilities in order to ensure a best outcome.

Post-surgery at the Hospital

You will be back on your feet before you know it. Current protocol is to get you up and moving as soon as possible. If you have anticipated this moment, you will be able to call upon what you have been learning immediately. As you stand up and put your feet on the floor again for the first time, you will be able to direct yourself into your length and balance and away from any possible pain.

Recovery is a process. Patience and persistence are essential. Take each stage as it comes, keeping the movement concepts you've learned in this book at the forefront of your mind. Take each stage as it comes. Work with it and watch the small shifts accumulate into real progress. As you stay with this process, you will see big changes without feeling like you have had to make any tremendous effort.

No doubt you will be working with a physical therapist. They too have their protocols and procedures. What has been presented in this book can complement any PT program. You can work with a physical therapist and attend to the AT principles simultaneously. You may need to move slowly at first. That is fine. Take your time. Your body has been reset and this is the ideal opportunity to further integrate your new habits.

The first of these new habits can be standing on both legs as evenly as possible. Do this each time you stand up from lying or sitting down. As you do this, sense your weight moving through your new hip into the ground and spreading out through your foot. Next, find your best balance on both feet. If you are using a mobility aid, make sure it is positioned to give you the most support and best connection into the ground. This will guide you to a better standing posture.

When you are ready, take a first step. Pause and take a moment to reset your balance on both legs. Recall the Movement Activities from Chapter 8 and continue to put in GAPs every few steps.

If you sense yourself compensating in any way due to pain or instability, put in a GAP. Pause on two feet until you feel balanced and only then, begin again. No shortcuts. Be sure to give this process the time it needs; it will serve you well.

Post-surgery at Home

The amount of time you spend in the hospital varies and depends on many things. It may be as little as 24 hours or as long as a few days. Regardless of how long your stay is, continue to work on your awareness while you are there. You will be so grateful you did once you are back at home.

Whether you have a lot of help once you are home or you are on your own, you will likely be thanking yourself for how much preparation you did to set yourself on the right track pre-surgery for your recovery. This applies not only to your new movement habits but also to how you have set up your environment and coordinated your social schedule. By having these things in place ahead of time, you will be able to handle whatever comes up.

Set up your own routine to include PT exercises, time on a passive movement machine, and icing. Make sure to allow time for recuperation. Also, be aware of trying to do too much or too little and adjust your prescribed activity level accordingly. It is important to use this time to review the concepts in this book. The more you can continue to work with them as part of your recuperation, the more complete your recovery will be.

Case Studies

I invited two Alexander Technique colleagues of mine, both of whom have had hip replacements, to share their stories. Their stories follow my own. I am struck by how similar our stories are and how the Alexander Technique played a part in all of our processes. I hope you find these stories interesting and helpful as well.

Ann's Story

I have been a very physically active person for my entire life. I ended up in the emergency room from cuts and lacerations multiple times a year until I was about 15 due to a hypermobile condition called Ehlers Danlos Syndromes. Each time, I recovered and ended up back to normal. My urge to move led me to study dance in school. My focus in graduate school was movement analysis and notation, which fed my interest in developing awareness as it relates to the body in space. As a dancer, I had the common aches, strains, and pains that come with that strenuous activity. I was fortunate to have had excellent dance instruction and to have found a few teachers who were also quite flexible. They helped me understand that going to the limits of one's range of motion isn't necessary, good, or in my case, even desirable. Stretching to the limit often braces and locks the joints, cutting off the flow of movement and making the small movements needed to maintain a refined balance impossible.

I was fortunate to discover the Alexander Technique during my years in graduate school at the Ohio State University. For nine years after graduate school, I taught dance in universities throughout the U.S. I, then, moved to New York City where I continued to choreograph and perform, and deepen my Alexander Technique practice.[6] I have been teaching the Alexander Technique now for over three decades. I am the founder and current director of the Balance Arts Center in New York City.

---

6   The Alexander Technique helped me organize the flow of movement and direct myself in a way that helped me find my overall dynamic balance. It helped me understand how one's body is meant to move and how I could embody those subtle principles and coordinations. Through thinking about how I was about to do a movement, not doing my normal pattern, and redirecting myself into better dynamic balance, I have come to an understanding of how to move with real ease and integration rather than just a loose body. This takes the pressure off my joints and, I have no doubt, saved me from many other problems that dancing with clEDS may have caused. While I was in graduate school, I made more technical progress once I started the Alexander work. I took fewer hours of dance class, paid more attention to how I was moving, and advanced technically.

Ehlers Danlos Syndromes (EDS)

I found out in my early thirties that I have a particular genetic connective tissue disorder called Classical Ehlers Danlos Syndromes (clEDS). This is one of 13 types of EDS. This discovery explained a lot. EDS can affect all of the connective tissue in the body, including skin, ligaments, heart, intestines—in short, every part of the body. It manifests differently in each person. In my body, clEDS partly manifested as easily stretchy and broken skin, which explains why I had had so many cuts throughout my childhood. I also experienced more than normal amount of flexibility, giving me a very large range of motion in all of my joints.[7]

My hyper-mobility turned out to be a mixed blessing. On the one hand, I can put my body in almost any position I choose, desirable in the circus and dance worlds. I used to be able to bring my leg up to my ear and also lie flat on the front of my torso while sitting on the floor with my legs out to the sides. I could do any basic pretzel stretch.

The downside of this hyper-mobility is there is so much play in the joints that there seems to be no limit or restriction to

---

7   A sense of fluidity and openness in the body and joints has always been part of my body awareness. That doesn't mean I always knew how to manage my movement. I had issues with stability and balance because I couldn't organize and coordinate a reliable postural system for support. At a sensory level, the sensation of being in one posture seemed to be equal to the sensation of being in another posture. There were few limitations to my movement.

movement. This means the basic integrity of a joint can easily be compromised. In my case, this happened with my left hip joint. Eventually, as the fluid in the joint capsule diminished and was absorbed into the bone, the bone of the pelvis met the head of my femur. Weight lifting, stretching, and the repetition of dance movements are contraindicated with EDS as they put extra pressure and strain on the joint tissues. This means that stretching can cause the myofascial system, including ligaments, tendons, and muscles, to lengthen more and more, further destabilizing the joints. With EDS, that tissue doesn't necessarily return to its proper tone, which potentially leads to further joint damage.

Although you may not have EDS and you might consider yourself tight and inflexible, principles of biomechanics, posture, and better functioning presented in this book still apply to you. Moving with instability has led me to focus on posture, alignment, and a way to move that doesn't cause further injury.

Not necessarily related to my EDS, I also have a grade 4 spondylolisthesis and slippage of one vertebra forward from the vertebrae below. Mine is at L5–S1 where L-5 is forward (anterior) to the normal alignment of the spine. L-5 was fused to S-1 from birth and makes it tiring to stand still for long. And I have a slight scoliosis, as most of us do. This seems important to mention as these conditions contribute to my overall balance and use. You, too, might have other conditions that factor into your recovery process.

Left Hip Story - First Signs of Concern

The deterioration of my left hip came on gradually over a period of about eight years. The first physical sensation I noticed was a twinge in the joint when pivoting on my left leg to make a sharp 90° right hand turn. The twinge evolved slowly into a sharp pain. At first, I assumed these twinges would pass in the same way other aches and pains had passed while I was dancing. Instead, I started experiencing stiffness in my left hip joint after sitting for a while. This was the first time I had ever been concerned about having a limited range of motion.

I developed a movement sequence combining yoga asanas, dance warm-up activities, and movements that felt good to do every morning and night to keep the hip limber and moving freely. Motion seemed to be the key to keeping my body lubricated and mobile, and, if I did the movement sequence regularly, I had almost all the range of movement I wanted.

Over the next three to four years, the twinge developed slowly into a dull ache. The beginnings of a limp came when I stood up from a long period of sitting. I had to stand for a moment, settle onto the ground, and then walk. I was used to dancing, teaching, and running around at will, so this was quite a change. I walked and continued with my daily move-ment sequences even as my overall daily activity was becoming increasingly diminished.

Then, for about a year and a half, I went through a very painful period. I could only walk for five minutes before I had to stand still or sit down for a moment. During that time, the range of motion in my hip joint was reduced so much that I couldn't lift my leg up off the floor at all while lying on my back. And I was definitely limping.

I was determined that pain and restricted movement wouldn't interfere with my work, daily activities, social life, or shrink my sphere of activity. I stopped wearing shoes with an elevated heel as they would cause both hips to ache. I tried not to make decisions about going out or completing a task based on my hip limitations. I realize now, post-op, that just having the inner dialogue about whether or not to get up to do anything was restricting.

I learned a lot about slowing down and not rushing. I started using handrails to go up and down stairs whenever possible. I gave myself extra time for outings to accommodate my slower pace. My friends were great about taking more time to walk with me and to wait for me when I needed to stop or sit down.

Looking for the root cause of the problem, trying to understand and figure out why this was happening is looking backwards. It is helpful to recognize what habits have been damaging. However, I know from my teaching that it is more productive to work with what is happening right now. The process of looking backwards can sometimes be extremely time consuming and, all the while, our habits of thought and use are still affecting us. Even when one knows the cause of the habit, the process for changing the current habits still has to take place. Our current habits come from many different sources (imitating our parents, copying the habits of friends or classmates, etc.) and life experiences (sports, injuries, emotional traumas, etc.). There is not necessarily a one-to-one correlation between a single event (except perhaps a specific accident or injury) and our movement patterns. The thoughts we think and the actions we take right now are the ones that will take us to a new and better functioning. Previous experiences and knowledge can and do inform our current movement choices. However, we need to continuously reinitiate and rethink how we are moving so we don't get stuck in a movement rut or develop a replacement habit.

My Movement Pattern Pre-surgery

My movement pattern before surgery was to hoist my chest off my legs and tilt my whole torso forward to try to make more space for movement and avoid the catching in my hip. I was very aware that I tilted forward in the torso much of the time. I looked physically heavier than I was because my body was not lengthened out. All of this exaggerated the twist I have in my spine and produced tension in my ankles, knees, hips, shoulder girdle, neck, and jaw.

Putting on my left sock and tying my left shoe were difficult tasks. My stomach muscles often spasmed and cramped on the left side when I did either of these things. I did better when I bent forward to touch my toes with my hands because I could mostly bend in my back rather than fold in the hip. After a while, even that type of movement made my abdomen spasm.

As a teacher of the Alexander Technique, I teach people to move with efficiency and coordination and I was concerned that I was not a good model for them. I was well-aware of my limp and general deteriorating movement long before I decided to have surgery. On some level, I still thought my hip pain would go away like all my dance injuries had and that I would be able to organize myself to think and function in an acceptable way in spite of the bone-on-bone connection between my femoral head and the acetabulum. After all, that is what I do for a living and what I teach others to do—think through how they are using themselves and allow the body to move as it is best designed to. I worked very hard to correct myself. I knew my hip should have been functioning a lot better than it was.

Real Trouble

The compensations finally caught up with me while I was on a trip, causing me to lie down for about an hour to let things settle. That was the turning point for me. I started searching for the right doctor.

I was not sure whether I was a candidate for a total hip replacement (THR), hip resurfacing, or some form of fluid injection into the hip. As I made the rounds to five doctors, it became fairly clear that a THR was needed. The bone-on-bone situation had caused cysts (cavities) in the head of the femur that compromised the integrity of the femur head, a resurfacing would be insufficient. I decided to go ahead with the THR, I wanted my hip pain to be resolved by a single surgery.

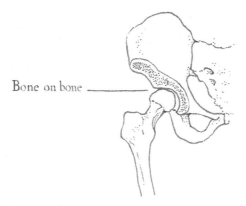

Fig. 18

Searching for the Right Doctor

The search for a doctor was a long-drawn-out, and challenging experience. I ended up seeing five doctors in all before making a decision. Finding the right surgeon took about six months and getting on the calendar for pre-op tests and surgery took several more months. I did not anticipate that once I finally admitted and surrendered to the fact that surgery was inevitable, it would take so long to organize.

When I started looking for a doctor, I wanted someone who was confident and skilled and had a good bedside manner. It was important to me that the doctor be open and curious with each patient and their unique experience.[8]

No doctor committed to just hip resurfacing, and they all hemmed and hawed over the option enough for me to know that the THR was the only real answer.

I was happy and fortunate to find Dr. Steven Stuchin from the New York University Hospital for Joint Diseases to do the surgery. He listened to me and understood my situation, both medically and professionally. Dr. Stuchin had done thousands of

---

8   I wanted to work with a doctor who would treat me as a person, believe my experience, be willing to entertain questions, and had expertise with clEDS. Each doctor was very different in his approach to assessing my situation. One shrugged his shoulders and did not understand there was a problem because I could go up and down the stairs to the subway and walk for as long as I wanted. Eventually he realized something needed to be done, especially after he looked at the X-rays and watched me walk.

hip surgeries and had experience with EDS. He was able to assess my situation rapidly and primed me well for what to expect. I sensed he was interested in my personal progress and recovery, and I saw him give all of his patients similar attention. He did an amazing job on my hip, for which I am extremely grateful.

Surgery

I was quite anxious before the surgery. I assume this is very normal. Turning one's entire body over to someone else to "fix" and reorganize it surgically is scary. It is definitely a journey into the unknown. Some people like to be put under with anesthesia, I am not one of those people. I have meditated for many years and was glad to have that as an anchor throughout the entire process. Even so, I had a fear of losing the leg completely during surgery.

Usually, the surgery is done with an epidural. However, after discussing my case with the anesthesiologist, we decided to use general anesthesia. This was due to the clEDS, which poses a potential risk of excess bleeding and spondylolisthesis. Also, my spinal fusion is where the needle for the epidural would typically be inserted. I was glad that we opted for general anesthesia, I didn't want to hear any of the sawing or pounding that I knew was going to take place.

Coming out of surgery was an amazing experience. Even as I climbed back out of the anesthetic fog, I knew my hip was better. It felt like my whole body had been reset and I could start anew with my movement habits. I was determined to do so. I was fortunate to not be in much pain which helped with my sense of possibility.

Post-surgery - Crutches to Walker to Cane

After my surgery, sitting up, taking weight on both legs, and walking for the first time was amazing. The previous limitations to my range of movement were gone and my left leg felt as if it could go anywhere. Dr. Stuchin said it might feel like I had a roller skate for a hip, and indeed, it felt amazingly loose and free. I had to be mindful, paying close attention to keeping the leg in line with the joint and not letting it wander. It felt as if I had no hip joint at all and my body just happened to fold in that particular location.[9]

It seemed as though the anesthesia "reset" my body and gave my muscular habits a whole new beginning. At least that is how I wanted to think about it. I wanted to drop the old patterns of compensation and develop new and better overall

---

9   I sensed my hip fold much lower and farther away from my head than I had for quite some time, pre-surgery. I know the anatomy of the hip joint from my work so my mental image is fairly accurate. Pre-surgery, though, my body couldn't allow a proper fold to happen. Post-surgery, I found that both legs could be closer together and more underneath me. One post-surgery precaution (having to do with the angle and location of the incision) involved avoiding crossing the body's midline with the legs to reduce the possibility of dislocation.

coordination with the new hip from my very first step. I moved slowly and deliberately with crutches.

On my first stroll around the hospital, I was able to walk around the floor (about 250 yards), moving from crutches to a walker after about 50 feet. And, I went up and down about five steps. From the start, I worked to use the crutches and walker as guides for finding my uprightness. By subtly intensifying a direction of up, back, and away from my hands, I could let the crutches take part of my body weight without collapsing and leaning on them. Leaning on them would only create a habit to be unlearned in the future, as I moved to a cane and ultimately to "hands-free" walking.

I was worried about taking my full weight on the new hip, but I was encouraged to do so. I thought the leg would wobble out of the socket, so I kept focusing on the leg going directly into the ground and coming back up into the socket. It also felt like I was going to walk forward out of the hip joint when my leg was even a little behind me—meaning the joint would pop out, if I stretched the front of the joint. Dr. Stuchin assured me that would not happen.[10]

The Physical Therapy staff at NYU-HJD were very helpful and supportive as they accompanied me around the hospital "track." It seemed like a track around the hospital because as my awareness expanded past my room following the surgery, I was aware that other patients who'd had hip surgery were doing their laps as well, each also challenging their limits in the process of rebuilding coordination and stamina. I became aware of which patient was passing by my room by the sound of their walker or crutches and the rhythm of their gait. It was enjoyable to witness everyone's progress and to hear their stories.

AT and My New Movement Life

My initial post-hospital recovery took place at a friend's house, where I was well taken care of. Each day brought more strength and coordination. I walked, rested, walked, rested, walked, and rested.

---

10   Cate, my friend, is a movement educator. She came to be with me during the surgery and was very helpful in giving guidance and feedback. She told me when I was limping, hiking up my right hip, moving with equal length steps, sinking onto the left or right hip, twisting, tilting forward with my torso, cross-patterning correctly, and so on. The new overall alignment was familiar to me from the past, before the compensations from the hip started, and still I needed to check in with someone to make sure my kinesthetic sensations were accurate. Matching reality with sensations can be a tricky thing, and I knew I needed to start putting the two together right from the start.

Soon, I was on my own walking around my loft in NYC. After two and a half weeks, I was able to return to the BAC and work several hours a day. By then, I was walking with a cane and sitting on an elevated seat while I worked.

I spent a lot of time walking slowly in my home space— monitoring how I moved and continuing to be vigilant about the movement precautions, restrictions to my movement given by the doctor. I have a big mirror for teaching and I walked forward toward it and then walked backwards away from it to monitor my gait. Walking backwards is a good activity for balance, to keep the feet limber, and allow the body weight to connect into the ground. I also checked to make sure I took equal step lengths, with each leg going forward as I did not want to build in any twisting in the hips or torso.

The most difficult and detrimental moments came when I attempted to walk quickly. When I did this, I lost my coordination, became disorganized, and reverted to hoisting myself along. I learned right away to walk at a pace where I could stay organized in terms of my use. When under stress of any kind, most of us tend to rely on a pattern that is familiar and that what we know will work, even if it isn't the best way to go about accomplishing the action. That was happening to me when I set off at too fast a pace.

6 Weeks Post-op

At the 6-week follow-up appointment, I was able to walk cane-free with only a slight limp. While I was aware that giving up the cane too soon could create patterns that would have to be unlearned, it was also clear that I had to let go of the cane as soon as possible. One of my students who had knee surgery about nine months earlier kept saying, "Get rid of the cane inside the house, get rid of the cane as soon as possible." She was right.

The actual moment of going "hands-free" was disorienting. At first, I had to talk myself into letting go of the support. I would walk with the cane for a few steps, then lift it off the ground to see what happened and how much I listed or collapsed in my body. I would go back to a few steps with the cane, doing the best I could with my gait, then let go again. Alternating between walking with and without the cane helped a lot.[11]

I continued to use the cane outside, mostly for safety purposes. The streets of NYC are crowded, and I lived near Ground Zero where there are many tourists unfamiliar with the

---

11   I can see how some might have to push through a few barriers to let go of the support of a cane, especially if there is even a small fear of falling. It could be very comfortable and secure to just keep the cane around all the time. I observe people on the streets walking with canes, but not using them. I always wonder why they have them—habit or necessity? Clearly, they feel more secure with them. It can be a big moment of trusting one's body and balance to let the cane go. I knew this moment was coming for me and I started walking short distances without the cane.

peripheral vision necessary to navigate the city streets. I wanted people to get the signal to be careful around me.

I was working to sense my body weight going into the ground through my new hip and whole body, to spread my feet out on the ground, and to allow my body weight to bounce back up through my body to give me a lift of lightness. I knew this works from all my Alexander Technique training. It is a very tangible sense of movement flow through the body that is both freeing and supportive.

It was tricky not to go for one specific "way" or "feeling" of moving just because it accomplished the goal of walking forward. From my Alexander training, I know it is important to both accomplish a task and look at "how" we are doing it. I know from my own experience how difficult it can be to change fundamental movement habits. That is why I spent so much time focusing on the "how." Once the "how" got sorted out the "what" of walking became so much easier. I wanted to walk fluidly and evenly while being upright. That meant I had to keep allowing the patterns to change and refine each time I went for a walk.

I was told that the first six weeks out of surgery would be the most dangerous time-period in the recovery process because that is when people feel better about moving and forget to be vigilant about restrictions on their range of movement, called precautions. I could see the truth in that. It was tempting to go on auto-pilot when moving around and just squat rather than lunge when picking something up. I was given permission to sit in any chair, take the booster seat off the toilet, and go out to dinner (oops, I did that already, carefully), but I had to continue observing the 90-degree or less rule of flexion for another six weeks.

I continued to check out my gait by watching myself as I walked slowly toward a big mirror. Some of what looked right felt wrong. In Alexander terms, we talk about this as unreliable sensory appreciation, when we have sensations that are inaccurate and need re-educating.

The visual guidance of the mirror was a tremendous help in assessing how I was doing. My kinesthetic sense told me I was leaving the right hip down as I walked forward. In the mirror, I could see it was definitely better than before, but there was more to go. This happened over and over again. The mirror doesn't lie. Doing more felt wrong, but the feedback I was getting from the mirror showed me I was moving along the right trajectory. There was always more to go and I had to let go of the physical sensations and focus on exaggerating the action and direction.

My new left hip was the most stable joint I had ever had in my body. I had never experienced the kinesthetic sense of joint stability before due to the clEDS. That stability allowed for an increased sense of direction everywhere else. The joint was tighter, meaning the femur fit more snuggly in the joint in a new way. I assume that is because Dr. Stuchin tightened the ligaments around the joint. The tiny screws he used to do that were visible on the X-ray. I began to sense a definite sinking into the right hip while I stepped forward onto the right leg. This was disconcerting.

Awareness of the kinesthetic sense, where your body parts are in relation to each other and to the surrounding space, is a curious phenomenon. A localized prominent sensation can dominate the whole bodily experience. A headache or toothache can dominate the whole field of awareness as can the pain of a restricted hip joint. There are always other things to notice that are not in ones field of awareness, and as my hip improved these other sensations started to surface.

I also know from my work with the Alexander Technique that the local site in the body where the attention is drawn is not necessarily the cause of the dominant sensation. I find that pain generally comes from the weak link or least integrated body part in the movement chain. This tends to be the place where the pressure builds up on the overall system. For instance, someone with a foot or knee concern may come in for a lesson. I always address the overall picture of the student's use and functioning before I address a specific area of the body or task that some-one wants to work on. I start with their head-neck balance and direction that brings the whole spine and torso along, too. Often a great deal of relief from the area of concern is experienced by the time there is dynamic whole body support.

Three-and-a-half Months Post-op

At a three-and-a-half month checkup with Dr. Stuchin, I was doing full squats and grand plies (And getting back up on my own, which was the astounding part), a plank (push-up position) with three points of support (lifting each leg up off the floor to the back), and balancing on each leg while bringing the opposite knee almost up to a horizontal level with the hip joint. And I was able to stand with my feet directly underneath me with my inner thighs touching. I could finally wash my feet without a long-handled brush and could tie my shoes comfortably. Before surgery, all of these movements had been off-limits.

In addition to restoring these physical capabilities, five pounds had dropped off by this time because I could walk more. I looked thinner in any case as my body had lengthened out. People said I looked younger (which is always nice) and many asked me if I had had a face-lift. Overall, my energy was great. All of those things let me know how much stress and strain had gradually crept into my body and whole being, prior to the surgery.

It amazed me how deep the compensatory movement patterns had become. I could tell at this point that the recovery process was not over. In fact, I was almost just beginning to recover. Now I was ready to move and explore what the new hip could do and how it could be a better part of my whole body picture.

Several years later I began having trouble with the other/right hip and could tell it was deteriorating in much the same way as the left hip had done. I had the second hip replaced 6 years after the first surgery. Because I knew what to expect with the surgical process, already had a surgeon I trusted, and knew how to manage the medical system, I started the hip surgery process much earlier than the first time around. I had a similar recovery period and was again fortunate to have friends around through the entire process. I was home within 48 hours of the surgery and had everything in place to rest and walk.

Now, after my two hip surgeries, I have taken tango lessons and moved on to other activities. I do a movement sequence and approach my old full range of motion gently. Walking is good. I continue to improve my movement every day as I work with the principles of the Alexander Technique.

Meg Jolley's Story

It is now April 2020. I am writing this recollection of my experiences with hip pain and bilateral hip replacements, with feelings of deep gratitude. I am thankful to have no pain at all in my hips or spine, and to enjoy fluid and full range of motion in my favorite activities of yoga, hiking, swimming, skiing and dancing. I appreciate recent invasive approaches in joint replacement surgery, which allow for minimal impact on muscles and tendons in the hip region, and structural materials that hold up well over time. I am grateful for the exhortations and expertise of activity and physio-therapists who helped me become stronger during months of pre-habilitative activity and weeks of surgery rehabilitation. The Alexander Technique has been the resource I draw on daily to support my recovered pain-free ease and freedom of movement, a resource that unfortunately is not standard protocol in the orthopedic community. Surgical advances and quality care through PT are important and available to all who undergo hip replacements. The addition of lessons in the Alexander Technique can potentially speed recovery time, promote a more even distribution of postural muscle tone which will minimize stress in the healing hip structure, and help people change long-held patterns of movement that may have contributed to painful erosion in the bones of the hip over time.

My own story is this: I have been a dancer all my life. Long-practiced stressors of jumping, and demands of balletic turn-out, coupled with a level of extreme flexibility, are integral to my own body-story. Uneven balance between postural stability and my own hyper-mobility has exacerbated structural wear and tear in my hips and knees over the course of my career. Arthritis runs through my family history as well. My own progression from occasional acute pain on weight bearing in certain positions—likely due to soft tissue damage and labral tears—to unavoidable debilitation caused by severe degradation of the bony architecture of my hips was years and years in the making. For some of that time, the Alexander Technique and disciplined attention to better use brought noticeable relief, but not recovery.

I was teaching Ballet, Anatomy and the Alexander Technique in a university when the pain in my right hip became chronic and quite excruciating, no matter how I might have marshaled my willpower, anatomical awareness, and Alexander Technique resources. The benefits of "good use" and efficient body mechanics were no longer possible for me, due to my overriding need to avoid pain. By this time, compensations of protective bracing had moved well beyond the territory of hips and legs, playing out through my whole body. As I look back on these months, I see myself moving through extreme discomfort, dissociation and fear. I was 59 years old, hobbling with a cane, trying mightily to avoid the extreme intervention of surgery. I was hobbled by fear, in equal measure to the pain.

Once colleagues, family, MRIs and orthopedic doctors helped me surrender to the idea that I would indeed have hip replacement surgery, once I stopped being ruled by fear, I began to move in a much more constructive direction.

For months, I worked closely with a Pilates/Gyrotonics activity teacher, who is now a colleague, friend and Alexander Technique teacher herself. Together we designed an activity program to target each of the muscles that cross the hip joint or support pelvic stability in any way. The intent was to bring these muscles out of "protection mode," to reawaken strength, mobility, elasticity and to promote better circulatory flow, before surgery. As a dancer, I found this program of countless leg-lifts, pelvic bridges and rotational "clams" incredibly mundane and mind-numbingly boring. Still, I am convinced that these months of pre-habilitative activity measurably improved my post-surgery recovery time by increasing resting muscle tone and bringing me to a higher "default setting" of strength and resilience in muscles that had been allowed to weaken and stiffen through lack of use.

When we are in pain, protection helps. I had been protecting, through minimal weight-bearing and restricted motion, for many, many months leading up to my surgery. The activity program I used for pre-surgery toning needed to be non-weight-bearing, repetitive, and within the limited range of mobility I could access without pain. So, lying on the floor, lifting my leg in seemingly endless repetitions, in all directions, and sustaining the hold beyond what felt aesthetically pleasing to a dancer was what I did.

The other valuable pre-habilitative practice was working out in a heated therapy swimming pool. Here, free from earth's gravity, I could walk in the warm water without pain, without protective patterns of pain avoidance, and sometimes with ankle weights to amplify the work-out. I could come back to my Alexander Technique use of direction in motion. I could move freely without pain, and even with joy again. Working in the water, whether with weights and an organized activity program, or running in deep water with a flotation belt, or simply free-form dancing without pain—all of these experiences, together with the targeted hip muscle strengthening program, prepared me well for my hip replacement surgery.

For the surgery itself, I was in the hospital for one day and one night, requiring pain medication on that first night only, with no need for pain meds at all after my release. I was up, walking, climbing stairs and ready to go home the day after the operation. My doctor has a video of me walking the halls of the hospital and waving my cane at him; he sometimes shows patients who are fearful of undergoing the surgery, as I was, this bit of video encouragement. I am not sure this is such a good idea—as I know the immediate recovery from hip surgery is not this "easy" for everyone. This is where the Alexander Technique has been invaluable for me. Having awareness of primary control, breath support, direction, allowing my head to lead and trusting my body to follow—all of the dearly held principles and practices we live with as Alexander Technique practitioners were readily available to support my recovery. My hip was no longer "human," and no longer generated pain. Walking, standing, rising from a chair, climbing stairs were once again activities I could bring myself to with awareness, inhibition, direction and delight. I moved slowly and carefully in those first weeks after surgery, exploring opening vistas of freedom and ease. I used the DART procedures with curiosity and intent to re-pattern movement coordination from the ground up. Working with Alexander Technique and the DART procedures helped me unwind from patterns of misuse that had been rooted in habits of protection from pain, and likely, before that, in my extreme mobility while dancing.

I enjoyed such a sense of ease, gratitude and relief in my recovery from this hip replacement that I did not procrastinate when labral tears and arthritic conditions in the left hip became more and more evident. Having had such a positive experience and uncomplicated recovery from my first surgery, I was (relatively) fear-free. Two years after my right hip replacement, I had the left hip replaced, with a similar course of pre-habilitative activity preparation and rehabilitative follow-up. My skilled orthopedic surgeon used a similar antero-lateral incision approach, which avoids cutting any muscle or tendon in the hip region. My recovery was once again, thankfully, smooth and uncomplicated. This time, because I was not so embroiled in hesitancy and fear, I was much more able to access my Alexander Technique practice throughout the months leading up to and immediately following surgery. To this day, now 6 years and counting past my last surgery, I am ever grateful for the sustaining practice of the Alexander work, as I stand here on my own two feet and my two bionic hips, allowing me to move through daily life free from the grip of joint pain.

Meg's Bio:

Meg Jolley, Movement Educator and AmSAT certified Alexander Technique teacher, has been on the Theatre/Dance Faculty at Pomona College for over 30 years. Currently, Meg directs the Movement Studies track of the dance major at Pomona. Through this program she offers both group and individual classes in the Alexander Technique, as well as courses in Anatomy/ Kinesiology, Somatic Movement, Experiential Anatomy and Mind in Motion. Meg also serves on the Board of Directors and Faculty for the Alexander Training Institute of Los Angeles and teaches privately in Pasadena and Malibu, California.

Pam Johnson's Story

I began having hip pain in my early 40s. I noticed it mostly at the end of long walks around my neighborhood. Walking on flat ground was worse than going up and down hills. I also started having pain during shopping trips at the local mall. I started planning my shopping trips around the location of rest benches! Ice became my daily friend.

I've been a mover my whole life. I was in dance classes at the age of 6. I was a baton twirler throughout my high school career (hey, I'm from Texas!), danced and performed in musical theatre in college, taught fitness and aerobics classes throughout my 20s and became a Pilates and Gyrotonic activity instructor in my 30s. Not being able to move well without pain was crippling physically, mentally and emotionally.

When my own "get out of pain" strategies weren't working any more, I decided to consult a hip and back orthopedic specialist. He diagnosed a herniated disk in my lower back and my hip pain as trochanteric bursitis. He prescribed physical therapy and suggested strength training in my core and hip muscles to relieve the pain.

Six weeks of physical therapy turned into several years, plus cortisone shots, acupuncture and chiropractic. I continued to have pain, especially when standing and walking. A spring break trip to Florida with my family was the final straw. I was in so much pain at the theme parks that I almost ordered a wheelchair. I had my doctor call in a prescription for pain meds to a local pharmacy. The meds helped, but I was a zombie for the rest of the trip.

After that painful vacation experience, I decided to research other solutions. My chiropractor suggested I get a second opinion from an orthopedist colleague she recommended who happened to specialize in knee injuries, not hips! He diagnosed the true source of my pain—congenital hip dysplasia! Together, we looked at my X-ray and it was very clear; my hip socket was too shallow. Then after an MRI, I received the exact diagnosis—bilateral hip dysplasia, moderate osteoarthritis with joint effusion and a large superior acetabular labral tear. My pain was primarily coming from the labral tear.

What is Hip Dysplasia? (from Mayo Clinic.com)

Hip dysplasia is the medical term for a hip socket that doesn't fully cover the ball portion of the upper thigh bone. This allows the hip joint to become partially or completely dislocated. Most people with hip dysplasia are born with the condition. Hip dysplasia can damage the cartilage lining the joint, and it can also hurt the soft cartilage (labrum).

At birth, the hip joint is made of soft cartilage that gradually hardens into bone. The ball and socket need to fit together well because they act as molds for each other. If the ball isn't seated firmly into the socket, the socket will not fully form around the ball and will become too shallow.

During the final month before birth, the space within the womb can become so crowded that the ball of the hip joint moves out of its proper position, which results in a shallower socket. Hip dysplasia tends to run in families and is more common in girls. The risk of hip dysplasia is also higher in babies born in the breech position and in babies who are swaddled tightly with the hips and knees straight.

Later in life, hip dysplasia can damage the soft cartilage (labrum) that rims the socket portion of the hip joint. This is called a hip labral tear. Hip dysplasia can also make the joint more likely to develop osteoarthritis. This occurs because of higher contact pressures over a smaller surface of the socket. Over time, this wears away the smooth cartilage on the bones that helps them glide against each other as the joint moves.

Diagnosis Made: A New Direction

Finally working with the correct diagnosis, I went on a quest to learn all I could about hip dysplasia, hip labral tears and how to live and function with this condition. I found an amazing website called Dancers' Hips. Through this site I got in touch with other movers and dancers who had similar hip conditions and had undergone various surgeries. It was an invaluable resource. I also consulted with two prominent orthopedic physicians specializing in hip arthroscopy. Was it possible to repair my torn labrum and return to pain-free functioning? Unfortunately, I was not a candidate for the procedure, due to my hip dysplasia.

During this same time period, I came across an *Introduction to the Alexander Technique* class being offered at my local YMCA. Out of curiosity, I signed up! The class was taught by Bill Plake, a gifted teacher and musician who I continued to study with for many years. During my first Alexander Technique active rest session or "lie down," I had an amazing release in my pelvis, lower back and sacrum. I was hooked for life!

As I continued my Alexander Technique study, I discovered postural habits and thinking patterns that were exacerbating my condition. The most prevalent were:

- Narrowing and over-arching my low back

- Lifting the front of my ribs

- Pushing my pelvis forward

- Tucking and over-squeezing my glutes

- Turning my feet out

- Constantly focusing on my hips and blaming everything on them

- Ignoring and pushing through pain

Through my deepening work with the Alexander Technique, my habits and compensations slowly began to unwind. Regular lie-down sessions were the key to calming my nervous system, allowing years of compensations to dissolve. However, my pain in weight bearing didn't go away. I desperately wanted the Alexander Technique to be the complete remedy to heal my hip joints. Although it didn't do that, it did create space in my mind and my body. I stopped over-reacting to my pain. I could do an activity with more ease and, most importantly, I could think more clearly.

As my 50th birthday approached, I was certain I didn't want to go through another decade of hip hell. I began interviewing Los Angeles area orthopedic surgeons who specialized in total hip replacement. One of those physicians suggested the option of a periacetabular osteotomy or PAO, where the hip socket is cut free from the pelvis and then repositioned so that it matches up better with the ball.

The PAO cuts the bone around the acetabulum that joins the acetabulum to the pelvis. Once the acetabulum is detached from the rest of the pelvis by a series of carefully controlled cuts, it is "reoriented" to a position that provides better coverage of the femoral head, thereby improving the stability of the hip joint and unloading the peripheral soft tissues. The acetabulum fragment is then secured with screws. This improves the coverage of the femoral head, decreases the instability associated with dysplasia, and unloads the peripheral labrum and articular cartilage.

The PAO option was attractive in that I would keep my own bone. However, it was extremely scary in that basically my pelvis would be "broken", and I would have a long road to recovery since both hips would have to be done. Plus, my age was a factor for whether the surgery would be successful. There were no guarantees that I wouldn't ultimately have to have a total hip replacement on both sides.

After more research and talking to patients who had undergone a PAO or a total hip replacement, I decided to have a total hip replacement of my left hip at Providence St. John's Health Center for Hip and Knee Replacements in Santa Monica, California. I was 47 years old.

I woke up from that first surgery with the thought, "Why is my left leg in a sling?" Then I remembered; I just had major hip surgery and it was over! Ah, I was relieved but also totally zonked from the anesthesia and apparently from too much blood loss. I had to have a blood transfusion so I could just sit up in bed. Once I stabilized, I was able to start moving pretty quickly with a walker and was home recovering on the fourth day after surgery. Two weeks later, I was walking with just a cane and then walking well on my own at six weeks.

Two years after my left hip replacement, my right hip became problematic. I knew it was coming but thought it would be much later. More tests and another diagnosis: right hip osteoarthritis with a superior acetabular labral tear and a paralabral cyst. I quickly decided to have a total hip replacement of my right hip. The surgeon performed an anterior approach hip replacement (my left was done with an anterolateral approach).

My overall recovery was easier with the right hip. During the surgery, however, my femur sustained a hairline fracture during the placement of the femoral stem. So, I only used partial weight bearing using crutches for three weeks. Once the crack healed, I was up and moving on my own with two new hips!

The Alexander Technique has been instrumental in my surgical recovery and in living with my bionic body! Before my experience with the Technique, I was trying to get the perfect alignment or the proper form of a movement so that it had a certain look or shape. I was also striving toward an unrealistic goal of getting my body back to a pre-pain performance level. Well, after two major hip surgeries, my body had new needs and new challenges. Once I accepted this reality, my movement practice began to change and grow in ways I never expected. Now, when I experience excess tension, fatigue or frustration, I allow myself time to rest, time to reflect, time for meditational movement with no rules, no judgment and nothing to get right.

I encourage anyone considering or recovering from surgery to explore a practice like the Alexander Technique to undo habitual compensation patterns, improve and relearn whole body coordination, and to relieve the stress of living with an injury and associated physical and emotional pain

Of course, I wish I had been born with perfectly formed hip sockets, but I now see my journey with hip dysplasia as a pathway to new opportunities and people that I might have never known.

Pam's Bio:

Pam has been a movement instructor and educator for over 13 years. She is an AmSAT certified Alexander Technique teacher and graduate of the Alexander Technique Institute of Los Angeles, completing a 3-year, 1,620-hour program. She is also a certified Pilates instructor with a certification from STOTT Pilates and is a licensed, certified GYROTONIC® Instructor. Pam uses postural re-education and mindfulness in action to help people of all abilities move with more ease, build strength without stress and flexibility without force. She also has a dance and theatre background with a Bachelor of Fine Arts in Theatre.

Pam Johnson, M.AmSAT Alexander Technique Teacher Certified Pilates and GYROTONIC® Instructor http://www. movewellwithpam.com

Using Mobility Aids

If you are using mobility aids or anticipate using them, this section is meant to reframe your understanding of how a mobility aid can assist you. Using an aid can be understood as a progression towards finding stability and balance, a process of moving from full or partial support to hands-free mobility.

Different mobility aids offer different kinds of support. When given a choice, you should experiment with your options to find the aid that works best for you. Crutches are most useful when one leg or the other must be non-weight-bearing. A walker, on the other hand, requires that you take some weight on both legs. A cane will probably be your last mobility aid before walking hands-free.

What follows is a discussion of how to use each of the mobility aids. First, read through all the directions for the aid you will be using. Then begin at the top, working step by step through the activity. Take your time and know that learning the proper use will allow you to progress more quickly.

You can further your progress as well if between each chunk, you insert a GAP, a moment of pause in which to re-find your balance. For a refresher on GAPs, you can review the discussion on chunked-up walking in Chapter 6 and the accompanying video #9.

Work at your own pace. In each GAP, think about:

- Sensing your whole body.

- Finding the ground and the GRF.

- Continuing to breathe.

- Sensing the space around you.

Using Crutches

While crutches are often prescribed in circumstances where you need to take no or minimal weight on one leg, they can also enable you to maintain your upright stance while allowing your body weight to be supported.

If you find yourself using crutches, the first step is to adjust them so they fit you properly. Once you have the right size crutches, you must set the hand grip to the height that is right for your body. That height will vary, depending on the proportions of your torso and the length of your arms. The ideal height allows your elbows to remain slightly bent when your palms contact the hand grips. Your armpits should not be touching the top of the crutches.

Once you have found the proper settings, you can work with the Movement Activity below to develop the strength and coordination to use your crutches well. As you work through the steps of this activity, study the accompanying images. Fig. 19 illustrates the proper use of crutches. Note how he maintains an upright stance, while the man in Fig. 20 collapses onto his crutches.

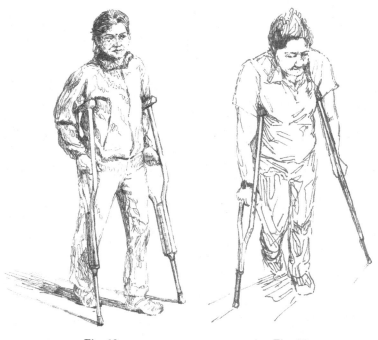

Fig. 19
Upright with Crutches

Fig. 20
Leaning on Crutches

Movement Activity
Crutches

(Video #20: Using Crutches)

Chunk #1: Set yourself up.

- With your arms outside your crutches, make sure there is space between your armpits and the top of the crutch pads.

- Check that your elbows are slightly bent, the palms of your hands placed easily on the handles.

- Let your back be long and your shoulders wide.

- If you are able, let your weight be distributed evenly on both feet.

Chunk #2: Move the crutches forward.

- Start by moving the crutches forward a little less than the normal length of your stride.

- Sense your weight almost simultaneously shifting to your more stable leg and into the ground through the crutches.

- Notice if you have hiked up your shoulders and allow them to release and be wide.

- Pause here and as much as possible, let your weight go into the ground.

Chunk #3: Prepare to step forward.

- Extend your free leg forward.

- Let the foot of your free leg contact the floor between the crutches. Keep your length so you stay as upright as possible.

- Pause and breathe fully into your torso allowing your shoulders to once again find their width.

Chunk #4: Step forward onto the front leg.

- Transfer your weight onto your front leg, allowing it to go into the crutches simultaneously.

- Bring your awareness to your palms on the handles and allow them to guide your sense of the counter direction occurring from the heel of your supporting foot to the top of your head.

- Allow this awareness to support you in staying long.

- Expand this awareness of your length to include your width—letting your breath be wide and deep and thinking of the loop that runs from your back through your elbows.

- Keep your head up so you can see where you are going.

Chunk #5: Bring your back leg forward.

- Bring the knee of your back leg forward while you support yourself on your front leg and the crutches.

- Step forward with the back leg, past your supporting leg.

- Take your weight forward onto your front leg by taking your head over that foot while you release the support of the crutches.

- Balance on this leg while you replace the crutches on the floor in front of you to start this process again.

- Return to Chunk #2.

Start by taking small steps and go slowly in order to build your coordination and stamina. Remember, the goal is to move with balance, ease, and coordination.

Using a Walker

At first, you may find yourself leaning on the walker and using it for substantial support. This is normal. When possible, the goal is to progress to using the walker for balance rather than support.

The Movement Activity below directs you in this transition. It is also useful in helping you transition from using the walker to using a cane. As you work through the steps of this activity, study the accompanying images. Fig. 21 illustrates the proper use of a walker. Note how she maintains an upright stance, while the man in Fig. 22 leans on his walker for support.

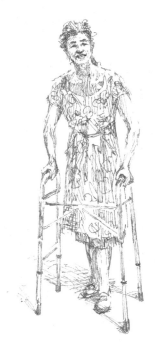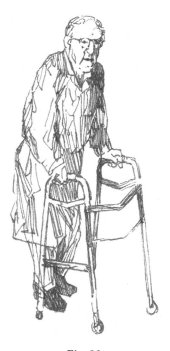

Fig. 21
Upright with Walker

Fig. 22
Leaning on Walker

Movement Activity
Walker

(Video #21: Using a Walker)

Chunk #1: Set yourself up.

- Start by standing inside the walker.

- Gently place your palms on the walker's handles.

- Adjust your weight so that it is evenly distributed on both feet.

- Make sure the walker is set high or low enough so that you remain upright when contacting the handles.

Chunk #2: Move the walker forward a short distance.

- Keep your torso as upright as possible.

- Balance on both feet.

- Roll the walker no more than 5 inches forward.

- Pause.

Chunk #3: Prepare to step forward.

- Shift your weight to your more stable leg.

- Allow your weight to go through that leg into the floor and rebound back up.

- Let your arms help you stay upright and balanced by thinking about coming up, back, and away from the walker's handles.

Bring your awareness also to the counter-direction occurring between your hands and head. Chunk #4: Fold your free leg.

- Next, let the knee of the free leg come forward toward the front of the walker, by allowing your hip and knee to fold until the foot comes only slightly off the floor.

- Pause.

Chunk #5: Step forward.

- Unfold the lower part of the free leg so that the entire leg extends forward.

- Let the heel contact the ground first.

- Keeping the walker still while taking your head over your front foot, allow your body to shift forward onto the front leg.

Chunk #6: Return to two feet.

- Fold the knee of your more stable leg.

- Allow that knee to come forward, unfold, and take your weight.

- Stand on both feet with your balance evenly distributed.

- Reinitiate your full height, thinking of the distance between the top of your head and the soles of your feet and vice versa.

Chunk #7: Take a second step forward.

- Stay up and back from the walker.

- Repeat this process, continuing to move forward.

- Work with this sequence until you can do it on both sides.

If at first you find yourself stabilizing mostly on one leg, notice this and use the above activity to refine your use. As you feel ready, start to experiment with using the other leg as your initial support.

From there, notice when you are able to stay upright as you scoot the walker out in front of you. Eventually, you will find yourself putting no weight on the walker at all. The goal, if and when possible, is to walk with your walker as if there is no walker. At this point, the walker has become a balance aid and you may be ready to progress to a cane.

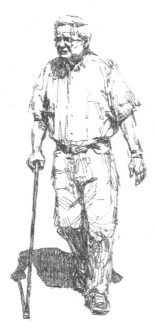

Fig. 23
Using a Cane

Using a Cane

A cane offers the least amount of support and the most freedom when it comes to mobility. For some, it will be the only device used while others will graduate to a cane from crutches and/or a walker. The cane can assist you in strengthening and refining your balance and can be used as long as it continues to be helpful.

Immediately arises the question of which hand should you hold your cane. Although it is optimal to use the cane on the side opposite from the one that needs support (in order to encourage cross-patterning), you may feel more supported when using it on the side that needs support (especially if it is your dominant side).

Because the cane is most effective when used for balance rather than full body support, the length of the cane is very important. When considering using a cane, take time to find a cane that is the right height. Ideally, when the cane meets the floor a few inches in front of you, your elbow should be slightly bent in order that the palm of your hand meets the cane's handle. The beginning of video #22 offers a visual guide to finding the cane height that is right for you.

Movement Activity
Cane

(Video #22: Using a Cane)

Chunk #1: Set yourself up.

- Start by finding your best upright stance, with the cane slightly in front of you.

- Adjust your weight so that it is evenly distributed on both feet.

- Place the palm of your hand on the top or handle of the cane, allowing your elbow and wrist to bend slightly.

- Notice how you have created a direct connection from your shoulder, through your arm to the cane, and on into the floor.

Chunk #2: Prepare to step.

- Maintain the full length of your body—from your head to the soles of your feet.

- Shift your weight onto your more stable leg.

- Initiating from the back of the knee, move the less stable leg forward until the foot of that leg is slightly off the floor.

Chunk #3: Prepare to step forward.

- Extend your free leg forward.

- Let the foot of your free leg contact the floor.

- Keep your length and stay as upright as possible.

- Pause and breathe fully into your torso allowing your shoulders to once again find their width.

Chunk #4: Step forward onto the front leg.

- Transfer your weight onto your front leg and into the cane simultaneously.

- Stay long from where the cane contacts the floor through to the top of your head.

- Allow this awareness to support you.

- Expand this awareness to include your width.

- Allow this sense of lift (what is, in fact, the GRF) to let you keep your head up so you can see where you are going.

Chunk #5: Bring your back leg forward.

- Initiating from the back of the knee, bring your back leg.

- Step forward with that back leg.

- Shift your weight forward onto what is now the front leg by taking your head over that foot and releasing the support of the cane.

- Balance on this leg while you replace the cane on the floor in front of you and start this process again.

Going Up and Down Stairs Using a Handrail

When it comes to going up and down stairs, the handrail is your mobility aid. All of the principles you have learned so far apply here as well.

Movement Activity
Going Up and Down Stairs

(Video #23: Going Up and Down Stairs)

Stepping Up

Chunk #1: Set yourself up.

- Stand at the bottom of the stairs with your weight evenly distributed on both feet.

- When possible, stand with your less stable leg next to the handrail.

- Place your hand on the handrail, slightly in front of your body.

- Let your back be long and your shoulders wide and easy.

- Place your more stable leg up onto the step in front of you.

- Sense your foot on the step as you move your arm forward up the handrail.

- Place your entire foot, if possible including your heel, on the step.

Chunk #2: Prepare to set up.

- Transfer your weight onto your less stable leg using the handrail for support, as needed.

- Remain upright with your head still above your supporting leg.

Chunk #3: Bringing your back leg up onto the step.

- Place your more stable leg up onto the step in front of you.

- Sense your foot on the step as you move your arm forward up the handrail.

- Place your entire foot, if possible including your heel, on the step.

Chunk #4: Step up.

- Think of the top of your head in relationship to the ceiling, allowing your body to lengthen into its full height.

- Shift your body weight up and forward over the front foot, sending your head away from your heel.

- Initiating from the back of the knee, bring your back leg up to the new step.

Chunk #5: Pause.

- Stand on both supports to re-establish your balance and posture.

Chunk #5: Repeat the process.

- Repeat this process with each step.
- Take your time.
- Allow yourself to refine the process with each step.

Stepping Down

Chunk #1: Set yourself up.

- Stand evenly on both feet at the top of the stairs.
- If possible, stand with your stable leg next to the handrail.
- Place your hand on the handrail, slightly in front of your body.
- Let your shoulders be wide and easy.

Chunk #2: Prepare to step.

- Transfer your weight onto your stable leg, using the handrail for support as needed.
- Keep your torso upright and long by coming up and away from the handrail.

Chunk #3: Place your less stable leg on the step below you.

- Lower your body weight by bending the knee of your more stable leg.

- Place the foot of your less stable leg on the step below.

- Use the handrail for support.

Chunk #4: Step down.

- Shift your weight forward and down onto your less stable leg as you let your arm slide down the handrail.

- Stay on your back leg as long as you need to, in order to transfer your weight smoothly onto the front leg.

Chunk #5: Step down.

- Bring your back leg down onto the lower step.

- Find an even stance on both feet.

- Re-establish your length.

Chunk #6: Repeat the process.

- Repeat this process with each step.

- Take your time.

- Allow yourself to refine the process with each step.

Once you have worked through the activities in this chapter and have progressed to using a cane, you will be ready to consider the possibility of walking hands-free. As you find yourself starting to use your cane less and less, refer back to Chapter 5 for activities that will help you reestablish your best gait.

Recuperation Strategies

Regardless of your physical condition, the work of changing and improving your movement patterns is very demanding. It is essential that you take time to recuperate in between activities. Actively resting serves as a reset that will allow you to continue with your activities with a renewed sense of balance and ease.

Below are activities and ideas you can use to reset yourself. Know that you can use them as often as you like. They will only help you to integrate this work more fully.

Lie Down

Doing an Alexander Technique Lie Down can be more restful than taking a nap. An active participatory process, it is an opportunity to organize the body using the least amount of muscular effort to support your system. Below is a simple guide. For a more detailed version, go to www.balanceartscenter.com and download the recording.

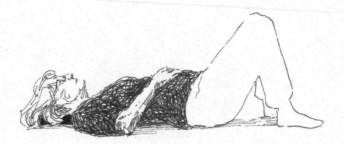

Fig. 25
Lie Down

Set yourself up for the lie down in one of the following two ways:

1. On your back, preferably on a firm surface. Lying on a
    mat or rug on the floor is best, however any firm sur-
    face works. If you haven't been down on the floor lately,
    you might want to start by lying on your firm bed or a
    massage table. Avoid anything like a couch, the surface
    of which is usually too soft, or any surface that slants in
    one direction or the other.

    Once you are horizontal, let your head rest on a paper-
    back book—or two, even three, depending on what
    you need to maintain the natural curve of your neck.
    Ultimately, as you lie there, your neck should be length-
    ened but not overly straightened and you should be able
    to breathe easily.

    During the lie down as your neck releases, you will
    feel the weight of your head going into the book more

completely. Stay easy in the tongue and jaw and continue to make sure you can breathe easily. As in Fig. 25, your knees are bent and the soles of your feet are contacting the surface you are lying on, so the weight of your legs does not pull on your lower back. Bring your awareness to the bottoms of your feet and sense your big toes connecting with the surface.

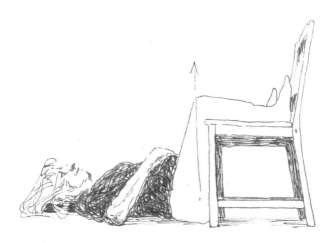

Fig. 26
Lie Down with Legs Up

2. If the first lie down option feels uncomfortable or you have difficulty keeping your knees directed towards the ceiling, you may prefer this second option with your legs on a chair. The added benefit to this alternative is that the weight of your legs goes directly into your hip sockets. You may find this more relaxing as it allows your pelvis

to release further. Note that, here too, your head is on a book or books, as needed.

Awareness Activity
Lie Down

Once you have organized yourself in the lie down that feels best for you, you are ready to actively direct your thinking to maximize the benefit of this activity. Below is a sequence of suggestions you can use to help continue building your awareness.

- Notice the places on your body that are contacting the supporting surface and let them soften.

- Sense the gravitational pull on your structure through those points of contact.

- Notice an upward rebound of energy and allow that to flow through your body.

- Bring your awareness to experience your full dimensionality.

- Let your breathing support that dimensionality and notice how the support is emerging from within your structure.

- Allow the dimensionality in your body to expand to include the space around you.

- Sense both your self and the space around you at the same time.

- Notice anything extra you might be doing or holding onto and let it go.

- As you do this, allow your sense of your whole body to increase, releasing further into your structure and the space around you.

The lie down is a practice. As you work with it, you will start to notice many other things. You may find moments of greater physical release, increased appreciation for the intricacies of your anatomy, the bond between mental and physical patterns, the ebb and flow of feelings, the shifting of your breathing, and much more. Let these experiences emerge and allow them to evolve. As you recognize them, watch them dissipate and de-intensify as they merge with your whole being and on into the space beyond.

The audio recording of a lie down (there are several, and one of them is available in multiple languages) can be found on the Balance Arts Center website. It takes you through a longer version of the practice and provides you with more specific suggestions.

The following activities, while not in the way that the lie down is, are critical aspects of a full and healthy mental and physical recuperation. They must be engaged with intentionally in the same way that you engage with your daily lie down practice.

Patience and Persistence

Post-surgery is a time that requires a balancing of three elements—the regaining of strength, recovering coordination and balance, and rest. Finding a balance between exertion and recuperation is a practice unto itself. You will have your own sweet spot and it will change daily. If your attention flags and you start mindlessly doing your exercises, it is time to stop and rest. And it is important to wait to resume your activity only when you can once again give your full attention.

If your muscles get so fatigued that you lose your form and best balance, the exercise will not be accomplishing its intended goal. It is best to take a break until you can reset and once again focus on *what* and *how* you are working. The more you resist going on automatic pilot and stay vigilant, the faster and more fully you will recover.

Stay in Touch

If you find that you are taking care of yourself alone, contact friends, family, colleagues and other sources of support on a daily basis. Whether in person or virtual, this contact with the outside world will make all the difference in your mood and ongoing motivation to recover.

It is best if you can have someone drop by once a day. If this is not possible, a phone call can be surprisingly uplifting and a reminder that you are cared for and matter. One word of advice: choose your company wisely. Connect with those who are supportive, encouraging, and interested in your progress.

Walking Buddies

Plan ahead for when you are really back up and walking. Before your surgery, line up your walking buddies. This way, they know to expect your call and you have something to look forward to.

Getting outside into the fresh air will feel incredible. At first, it may be as simple as walking to the corner or around the block. These accomplishments will be huge and should be celebrated. They are a first step in expanding your world back to its normal range.

You will be walking more slowly than you were used to pre-surgery. Let this be okay and use it as an opportunity to explore in more detail the world around you. You may be surprised at what new things you notice in what are otherwise very familiar surroundings. And if you have a park nearby, head over there as soon as you feel ready.

Practical Pre- and Post-Surgical Tips

Pre-surgery

Anything you do to prepare before your surgery will help ease your mind and allow you to fully focus, post-surgery, on healing and recovery. In addition to the pre-surgery movement activities in Chapter 5, you can work with these ideas:

- Take the time you need to find the right doctor.

- Make a list of questions. Be sure to write them down and take them with you to your appointment.

- Take notes at the appointment.

- Take someone with you to your appointments who will help you remember to ask all of your questions, take notes, and help you consider the answers afterwards.

- Know that once you decide that surgery is necessary and have found the right doctor, you will probably have to wait three to six months for the actual surgery.

- Use assistive devices, like a cane, earlier than you might feel is necessary to reduce compensations in the rest of your body.

- Prepare your house before you go into the hospital, making it easier once you return home to observe any precautions or movement restrictions given by your doctor. Invite a friend or family member to be at the hospital with you during the surgery so you see a familiar face when you come out of the anesthetic haze.

- Organize music or reading material for your time in the hospital. Even though your stay may be short, it will be helpful to have something to do.

- Organize your transportation home from the hospital.

- If you live alone, line up people to stay at home with you for the first few nights, so you feel safe and cared for.

Pre-surgery at Home

- Pull up rugs and any trip hazards.

- Stock up on food and supplies.

- Organize the delivery of groceries and supplies.

- Make sure you have cash on hand.

- Do your laundry.

- Clean your house.

- Prepare the tub or shower with a booster seat and hand grips.

- Make sure there is a non-slip surface in your shower or tub.

- Have extra pillows and props to support yourself in bed and on the couch.

- Elevate your bed so you can get in and out more easily.

- Find out what identification you will need at the hospital.

- Find out if you have any co-pays that will need to be paid at the hospital.

- Have your health proxy organized.

Post-surgery

Here are some practical things to consider immediately after surgery. These may seem like they have nothing to do with hip health and the Alexander Technique. Knowing these details are taken care of, however, will free you to focus fully on your physical recovery.

- Don't hesitate to take pain medications as recommended. Staying ahead of the pain allows you to relax, which accelerates healing.

- Ask for help as needed.

- Get up and walk as often as you are asked to. The sooner and the more you walk, the better.

- Take advantage of this time to rest and sleep as much as possible.

- Treat yourself by having someone bring you food from outside the hospital.

- Be sure to have someone other than yourself available to advocate for you.

- Enjoy your roommate, if you have one.

- Consider moving into rehab, if you are offered the opportunity. The personal attention can help accelerate your recovery.

- Thank the nurses, physical therapists, and hospital staff, often. You'll be amazed at how good this makes you feel and believe it or not, connected with your own body.

- Encourage friends to visit and check in with you as often as possible.

The Alexander Technique
at the Balance Arts Center

The Balance Arts Center is dedicated to teaching mindfulness and awareness in action through the principles and practices of the Alexander Technique. At the BAC, we teach awareness in action in private lessons, group classes, specialized workshops & conferences, and Training Programs. Founded in 2008 by Ann Rodiger, the BAC is now in its largest location, in midtown Manhattan, New York City, equipped with a performance space and state-of-the-art teaching and practice rooms. The BAC offers programming based in the Alexander Technique online and in person.

Offerings include:

- Programming for new students, wellness seekers, those interested in better posture and/or recovery from injury, and performing artists
- Private lessons in the Alexander Technique

- Programming for those with hypermobility

- Performing Arts Certificate (300 hours)

- Alexander Technique Teacher Training Course (1600 hours)

- Continuing Education (CTLE) credits for New York State Public School Educators

- Student Visa program for students at the Balance Arts Center

All teachers and faculty of the Alexander Technique who teach for the Balance Arts Center have graduated from a rigorous 1,600-hour teacher training program. All BAC teachers are certified through the American Society of the Alexander Technique or an Affiliate Society. The BAC faculty teach in NYC and around the world.

For more information visit: www.balanceartscenter.com

Contributing Influences

F.M. Alexander's story is useful and important in that it provides us with a process for awareness building, discovery, and change. His understanding of movement and flow came from his self-awareness and movement observations when he lost his voice while engaged in public speaking.

One of the most important aspects of Alexander's journey was that he understood how much he could, through his own focused thinking and practice, change his vocal use. His goal was to be able to speak in a theater without losing his voice. Doctors verified that his vocal anatomy was working properly. However, he recognized it was the way he was coordinating his breathing and phonation processes that interfered with his vocal ability. He spent time in front of mirrors assessing his own posture and the use of his body in a detailed way until he identified how he was hindering his vocalization. He worked with his posture to sort out his patterns of interference and replaced them with better balance and alignment.

In addition to the teachings of F.M. Alexander, the discoveries and teachings of Rudolf Laban, Raymond Dart, and Irmgard Bartenieff have significantly contributed to my movement philosophy and informed the content of this book. I would like to take a moment to introduce you to them as well.

The work of Rudolf Laban (1879-1958) offers a way of observing and organizing movement that provides vocabulary for the "what, how, shape, and spatial orientation"[12] of the body in motion. Movement of any sort and from any culture can be seen through the Laban lens. Laban's way of analyzing movement has been applied to personality assessment, human movement development, choreographic exploration, movement recording and documentation, industrial movement efficiency, and cross-cultural research.

Raymond Dart (1893-1988) was an Australian anatomist, doctor, and anthropologist. He is best known for his discovery of the *Tuang Child*[13] in South Africa. Dart's discoveries

---

12 Laban gave language to help us observe, describe, and document the various aspects of human movement. He developed **Labanotation** to represent the *what,* **Effort** to describe the dynamics and qualities of *how,* **Shaping** to describe *how* the body changes shape, and **Choreotics** (spatial theory) to define the space. These theories were further developed by Lisa Ullman, Irgard Bartenieff, Warren Lamb, Judith Kestenberg, and others.

13 Dart discovered the fossilized skull known as the Taung Child in 1924 at a Limestone Quarry in South Africa. It is the skull of an extinct species that lived approximately 2 million years ago. This discovery has been called "the most important anthropological ossi of the twentieth century" by Dean Falk, a specialist in brain evolution.

on the origins of human uprightness would play out on a personal level for him when he eventually became the parent of a brain damaged child who had difficulty standing upright and walking. Beginning in 1943, Dart developed a series of movements, called the Dart Procedures, to help his son work with his spasticity. Dart's work attracted the interest of Alex and Joan Murrray who introduced the procedures to the Alexander Technique community.

Irmgard Bartenieff (1900-1981) was a physical therapist, dancer, and choreographer, with expertise in movement analysis. She was a student of Rudolf Laban and incorporated his theories in her movement analysis and in the creation of the Bartenieff Fundamentals, which were first developed to aid people suffering from polio. Her sequences can assist anyone in developing basic movement coordination.

REFERENCES

Video Catalog

Chapter 1

#1: Hi-bounce ball and Bean Bag (page 24)

This activity explores gravity and the ground reaction force. It will help you sense the rebound in the ground reaction force that you can experience in your body. You will need a ball and a bean bag (or a book).

#2: Dynamic Balance (page 27)

In this activity you are going to see and experience how small movements of the eyes and head (moving parts) affect the balance of your whole body

#3: Compensations (page 31)

This activity helps you notice what happens to one part of your body while another part of your body moves out of alignment or has a restricted range of motion.

Chapter 2

#4: Head and Neck (page 36)

This activity shows you the head on the spine and how the head moves.

#5: Head, Neck, and Back (page 38)

This video shows you how to explore your head, neck, and back.

#6: Arms (page 41)

This video shows you how to explore your arms.

#7: Legs (page 46)

This video shows you how to explore your legs.

Chapter 3

#8: Hip Joint (page 52)

This activity guides you to explore your own hip joint to see where and how it can move. You will identify the body landmarks and see a video of a pelvis in motion.

Chapter 6

#9: Walking (page 73)

Chunking up walking is useful so that you can explore each element of the step. You can then redirect by putting in GAPs at critical moments.

Chapter 8

#10: Small Movements (page 112)

This video guides you through a number of small movements that will help you get back into moving. They are especially helpful if you haven't been moving for a while.

#11: Moving Your Torso from Both Ends (page 114)

This activity helps you discover both ends of your torso and the space in between the two ends.

#12: Rolling Down, Rolling Up (page 116)

This activity helps you to find mobility, flexibility, and coordination in your head, neck, and back, and integrates movement throughout your entire spine.

#13: Roll Down with Torso Extension (page 117)

This activity continues to lengthen and coordinate the entire head, neck, and back. Any amount of curl and extension can be helpful.

#14: Seated Spirals (page 119)

This activity integrates movements of your head, neck, and back with looking, turning your head, and the spirals throughout your torso.

#15: Re-establishing Your Balance (page 120)

This exercise will help you discover and refine your starting balance for all of your activities.

#16: Wall Push-ups (page 122)

This activity will help you find the full length of your body, head to feet, and refine your balance. You will also integrate your arms with your head, neck, and back, while taking minimal weight on your arms. You are effectively on all fours (two feet and two hands), while you are vertical.

#17: Walking in Place (page 124)

Walking in place helps you focus on and refine the movement of your legs without movement through space. It is good practice for the coordination of movement from one support to the other.

#18: Sit to Stand – Stand to Sit (page 126)

Spending time refining how you sit and stand is important for your recovery and future movement-related activities. It is an action most of us perform many times a day without thinking. Bringing these actions in to deliberate focus will help make them easier and more balanced

#19: Balancing on One Leg (page 128)

Each time you walk, you are balancing on one leg for part of the time. Practicing balancing on one leg will help you with more ease and overall balance.

Appendix I

#20: Using Crutches (page 178)

Using your crutches as a support for balance is important. They can help you regulate your weight as it moves through your new hip, while you improve your overall posture.

#21: Using a Walker (page 182)

Using your walker well will set you up for moving more easily to a cane. When you use your walker well, your balance and posture can improve.

#22: Using a Cane (page 187)

Maximizing the use of your cane is important. A cane is not something to lean on but rather a stability support to help you find your best balance.

#23: Going Up and Down Stairs (page 190)

Going up and down stairs can require a special choreography while your hip is recovering. Learn how to negotiate the stairs in the easiest way possible.

References:

Alexander, F. Matthias. *Constructive Conscious Control of the Individual.* 3rd ed. London: Mouritz, 2004.

Alexander, F. Matthias. *Man's Supreme Inheritance: Conscious Guidance and Control in Relation to Human Evolution in Civilization.* 6r.e. ed. London: Mouritz, 1996.

Alexander, Frederick Matthias. *The Universal Constant in Living.* 4.r.e. ed. London: Mouritz, 2000.

Brennan, Richard. *The Alexander Technique Manual: Take Control of Your Posture and Your Life.* London: Eddison, 2018.

Calais-Germain, Blandine. *Anatomy of Breathing.* Seattle: Eastland, 2006.

Carrington, Walter. *Thinking Aloud: Talks on Teaching the Alexander Technique.* Berkeley, CA: Mornum Time, 2002.

Clear, James. *Atomic Habits: An Easy & Proven Way to Build Good Habits & Break Bad Ones.* New York, NY: Avery, 2018.

Coyle, Daniel. *The Talent Code: Greatness Isn't Born. It's Grown. Here's How.* New York: Bantam, 2009.

Dewey, John. *How We Think.* London: D.C. Heath, 1909.

Ericsson, Anders, and Robert Pool. *Peak: Secrets from the New Science of Expertise.* Boston: Mariner /Houghton Mifflin Harcourt, 2017.

Fehmi, Les, and Jim Robbins. *The Open-Focus Brain: Harnessing the Power of Attention to Heal Mind and Body.* Boston, MA: Trumpeter, 2007.

Gelb, Michael J. *Body Learning: An Introduction to the Alexander Technique.* 2nd ed. New York: Holt, 1992.

Gendlin, Eugene T. *Focusing.* Toronto: Bantam, 1982.

Gilroy, Anne M., Brian R. MacPherson, and Lawrence M. Ross. *Atlas of Anatomy.* Stuttgart: Thieme, 2008.

Gordon, J. E. *Structures: Or Why Things Don't Fall Down.* Cambridge, MA: Da Capo, 2003.

Gorman, David. *The Body Moveable: Blueprints of the Human Musculoskeletal System - Its Structure, Mechanics, Locomotor and Postural Functions.* Ontario: Learning Methods Publications, 2002.

Gray, John. *The Alexander Technique.* New York: St. Martin's, 1991.

Hackney, Peggy. *Making Connections: Total Body Integration Through Bartenieff Fundamentals.* New York: Routledge, 1998.

Hall, Edmund T. *The Hidden Dimension.* Garden City, N.Y: Anchor, 1969.

Jones, Frank Pierce. *Freedom to Change: The Development and Science of the Alexander Technique.* London: Mouritz, 1997.

Kamhi, Ellen, and Eugene R. Zampieron. *Alternative Medicine Definitive Guide: Reverse Underlying Causes of Arthritis with Clinically Proven Alternative Therapies.* 2nd ed. Berkeley, CA: Celestial Arts, 2006.

Kapit, Wynn, and Lawrence M. Elson. *The Anatomy Coloring Book.* 4th ed. New York, NY: Pearson, 2013.

Laban, Rudolf. *Choreutics.* Alton: Dance, 2011.

McCredie, Scott. *Balance: In Search of the Lost Sense.* New York: Little, Brown, 2007.

McLaren, Galloway Niall T. *Seeking Symmetry: Finding Patterns in Human Health.* Edinburgh: Handspring, 2018.

Murray, Alexander. *Alexander's Way: Frederick Matthias Alexander, in His Own Words and in the Words of Those Who Knew Him.* Seattle: Seattle, 2015.

Myers, Thomas W. *Anatomy Trains: Myofascial Meridians for Manual and Movement Therapists.* Edinburgh: Churchill Livingstone, 2014.

Pallasmaa, Juhani. *The Eyes of the Skin: Architecture and the Senses.* London: John Wiley and Sons, 1996.

Perry, Jacquelin, and Judith M. Burnfield. *Gait Analysis: Normal and Pathological Function.* Thorofare, NJ: Slack Incorporated, 2010.

Phillips, D.C, and Jonas F. Soltis. *Perspectives on Learning.* New York: Teachers College, 2009.

Sacks, Oliver. *A Leg to Stand On.* New York: Touchstone, 1998.

Sobotta, Johannes. *Atlas of Human Anatomy.* New York: G. E. Stechert, 1930.

Strozzi-Heckler, Richard. *The Anatomy of Change: A Way to Move Through Life's Transitions.* Berkeley, CA: North Atlantic, 1997.

Vineyard, Missy. *How You Stand, How You Move, How You Live: Learning the Alexander Technique to Explore Your Mind-Body Connection and Achieve Self-Mastery.* Cambridge, MA: Da Capo Press, 2007.

Wheeler, Sharon L., and Jan E. Trewartha. *Scars, Adhesions and the Biotensegral Body: Science, Assessment and Treatment.* East Lothian, Scotland: Handspring Limited, 2020. Print.

Zander, Rosamund Stone, and Benjamin Zander. *The Art of Possibility: Transforming Professional and Personal Life.* Camberwell, Vic.: Penguin, 2002.

Key Concepts

The following are key concepts we work with in the Alexander Technique at the Balance Arts Center. They have been woven into the content throughout this book. It is also useful to look at each concept separately.

Alexander Technique: The Alexander Technique is a mindful process for building and increasing awareness of your sensory experience as it integrates with your thoughts. Cultivating awareness then gives choice and options—in action, thoughts, and emotions—in response to internal and external stimuli.

Attitude toward learning: An attitude of curiosity and discovery opens the door to new possibilities and growth. Opening our minds and bodies to exploration of what is, challenges what we think are fixed habits and ideas and allows us to make different choices and have new experiences.

Attention: Paying attention means noticing and attending to your thoughts and sensory experiences. It means directing your awareness to the present moment and your experiences in the now.

Biotensegrity: Dr. Stephen Levin, who coined the term biotensegrity, applies the concept of tensegrity to the structure of the human body and other biological structures. In this paradigm, there is a dynamic balance of push and pull forces throughout the bones, ligaments, fascia, and other tissues that creates a suspended structure.

Choice: Having the capability to choose from different options in thinking and movement. In practice, this is when we allow ourselves to make new choices in movement rather than go on auto-pilot and into our habit.

Chunk: "Chunking" is segmenting a movement or phrase of movements into discrete sections that can be examined and experimented with on their own. Once we finish working with chunked-up sections, we can put them back into the larger movement.

Counter Direction: This is flow that moves in two directions at once, e.g. up and down, out and in, side to side, front to back.

Direct or Directing: Giving yourself ideas to think about that apply to your body's movement and relationship to your environment, such as unlocking your knees, sensing gravity underneath you, and keeping your peripheral vision.

Direction: Direction is the literal spatial pathway through your body. It extends out into space around your body as well. Many of the ideas in this book include directions such as the Ground Reaction Force (GRF) moving from the floor up through your body and out the top of your head.

Dynamic Balance: Allowing your body mechanics and musculature to adapt to what is needed in the moment for optimal balance and flow in the structure. This means your joints are available to move and your musculature is available to adjust its tone as necessary to accomplish an activity.

Flow: The movement and energetic force that moves through your structure. We can experience flow, cultivate it, and allow it to support us in our movement. Our structure supports us in experiencing flow when we get out of the way, meaning when we stop holding ourselves together or thinking we have to "do" something extra to maintain our form.

GAP: A moment in a movement when you **GIVE A PAUSE**, regain your best balance and flow, and then move from there. The GAP is a way to inhibit your habitual pattern of thinking and moving, so you can make a new choice.

Habit: Our automatic and habitual response to a stimulus. The stimulus can be internal or external. When we consistently have the same response to a stimulus, we have formed a habit. Our goal is to cultivate a habit of choice in order to facilitate our constant change and growth into a greater sense of ease and expanded sensory experience.

Kinesthetic Sense: This is the sensory experience of movement of a body part or segment in relation to other body parts or segments.

Posture/Alignment: Posture and alignment are the relationship of the parts of your body to each other. Remember "good" posture is not a shape or held position, but a relationship of parts that is dynamic and adaptive to the requirements of the moment.

Rebound: The flow of our body's gravitational force, what gives us the sense of Ground Reaction Force (GRF) or upward direction. Tuning into the rebound as it flows through our bodies makes way for a sense of lightness and suspension throughout the entire system. In order to experience rebound, we have to take away any interference or blockages in our body's response to gravity and the GRF, meaning releasing any excess tensions or collapse patterns that stop the flow.

Redistribution of Tone: When movement patterns change, the tone in the musculature can also change to accommodate new movement habits. As the new pattern becomes familiar, the muscular tone will rebalance. Some muscles will be recruited while others will diminish their tone. There is always some tension or tone in the body. Our goal is to use the musculature necessary to do only the work needed in the moment.

Release into your "Directions": Allow yourself to let go of any excess tension you might be holding and let the energy from that holding go into your length, width, and depth, so you can connect with the (GRF) more clearly.

Spatial Intention: Deliberately perceiving and thinking of internal and external space, directions, dimensions, and volumes, in and around us. This gives us support for ourselves and perspective on our movements, our thinking, and our actions.

Throughness: An equestrian term that refers to the rider sensing the ground "through" the horse's body. When this concept is applied directly to the human body, we can understand it as sensing the pathways through the body that allow us to experience the oppositional gravitational forces, down and up, simultaneously. In order to experience thoroughness we want to remove anything that interferes with the gravitational flow.

Unified Field of Awareness:

Use: The manner or way in which we coordinate and manifest our movements, the way we function. Our habits and thought processes help determine our use.